SELECTED READINGS IN ACUMOX CLASSICS

Editor-in-Chief

Wang Jing

Shanghai Scientific & Technical Publishers

图书在版编目（CIP）数据

针灸经典选读 ： 英文 / 王静主编． -- 上海 ： 上海科学技术出版社，2025．7． -- ISBN 978-7-5478-7191-1

Ⅰ．R245

中国国家版本馆CIP数据核字第2025067HR5号

SELECTED READINGS IN ACUMOX CLASSICS

Editor-in-Chief　Wang Jing

上海世纪出版(集团)有限公司
上 海 科 学 技 术 出 版 社　出版、发行
(上海市闵行区号景路159弄A座9F-10F)
邮政编码201101　www. sstp. cn

开本 787×1092　1/16　印张 12.25
字数 300千字
2025年7月第1版　2025年7月第1次印刷
ISBN 978-7-5478-7191-1 / R·3289

About the Book

Selected Readings in Acumox Classics is an acumox literature textbook based on the teaching practice of acumox literature courses of Shanghai University of T.C.M. Taking into account the characteristics of the subject, the audience, the needs of students, *Selected Reading in Acumox Classics* employs the principle of "classification and selection" to emphasize the theoretical framework and evolution of acumox theory. That is to say, it categorizes and selects original texts related to important theories on meridians and acupoints, acupuncture and moxibustion, and acupuncture therapeutics from historical literature, particularly those with significant differences in meaning between ancient and modern times. These documents are analyzed chronologically, from ancient times to the present, to compare their evolution. The topics covered in this book include meridians and collaterals, Yuan-source points, reinforcing and reducing in acupuncture techniques, Deqi, the heat syndrome and moxibustion, and cold, heat, deficiency and excess in treatment principles of acupuncture and moxibustion.

Since the 1970s, the discovery of acumox documents and cultural relics in places such as Mawangdui and Zhangjiashan has revealed that the origins of acumox can be traced back to periods before *The Inner Classic*. Consequently, our understanding and development of acumox theories can no longer be solely based on *The Inner Classic*. Moreover, modern acumox works, especially those from the Republic of China period, played an important role in the modernization of acumox and are an essential component in the development of acumox theory. Therefore, the literature coverage of *Selected Readings in Acumox Classics* spans from the silk books predating *The Inner Classic* to the Republic of China era.

This textbook can be utilized for various forms of international acumox education and is also suitable for bilingual acumox teaching for Chinese students. For acumox practitioners who use English, this textbook serves as a reference work to explore the development of acumox.

Editors' List

Editor-in-Chief

Wang Jing
Shanghai University of Traditional Chinese Medicine

Associate Editor

Li Lei
The University of Hong Kong

Editorial Board Members

Zhang Chao
Shanghai University of Traditional Chinese Medicine

Hu Li
Shanghai University of Traditional Chinese Medicine

English Language Editor

Zou Qi
Shanghai University of Traditional Chinese Medicine

Introduction

With the growing popularity of acupuncture and moxibustion ("acumox[1]") and the advancement of its theoretical research, the importance of ancient acumox literature for the development of this field has become increasingly recognized. In this context, courses on ancient acumox literature are being incorporated into English-taught TCM programs for international students in higher education. Compared with other acumox courses such as Meridians, Acupoints, Acumox Techniques, and Acumox Therapeutics, there are very few English textbooks available for ancient acumox literature courses; and in Chinese textbooks for such courses, acumox literature is typically categorized into two major groups: classics written before the Eastern Han Dynasty (i.e., *The Inner Classic* and *The Classic of Questioning*), and various medical works written after the Wei and Jin dynasties. Common textbooks usually summarize the contributions of the original works, select or excerpt the original texts by chapter, and arrange them in the order of the original book. The main difference between the Chinese textbooks used at our university and other textbooks is the "categorization and selection". Specifically, the excerpted medical texts in our textbooks are classified and arranged according to meridians, acupoints, acupuncture techniques, etc., rather than following the order of the original works. For later medical works, summaries classify and explain the contributions of the original work according to meridians, acupoints, acupuncture techniques, etc. However, in many cases, the original texts cannot be easily classified due to the limitations of the content.

The purpose of studying ancient acumox literature is to trace the development of acumox theory, clarify its origins, deepen our understanding of acupuncture theory, and strengthen the links between acumox literature, clinical practice and basic research. The original Chinese acumox literature course

1. Acumox: Acumox is an informal and not widely accepted abbreviation of acupuncture and moxibustion. Acupuncture may be used to refer to both acupuncture and moxibustion, but this may cause some misunderstanding in certain contexts where moxibustion should be regarded as an independent therapy. The full term of acupuncture and moxbustion is too long, so in this book, this informal acumox will be used to refer to this term.

model can certainly achieve this goal. However, international students might face significant challenges due to limitations in language proficiency, cultural background, and cognitive styles, which may exceed their current capabilities. Taking into account the characteristics of the subject, the audience, the needs of students, and the specific features of our university's acumox literature courses, *Selected Reading in Acumox Classics* utilizes a model based on our university's Chinese textbook. It employs the principle of "classification and selection" to emphasize the theoretical framework and evolution of acumox theory. That is to say, we categorize and select original texts related to important theories on meridians and acupoints, acupuncture and moxibustion, acupuncture therapeutics and other important topics from historical literature, particularly those with significant differences in meaning between ancient and modern times. These documents are analyzed chronologically, from ancient times to the present, to compare their evolution. In addition, since the 1970s, the discovery of acumox documents and cultural relics in places such as Mawangdui, Zhangjiashan, Shuangbaoshan, Laoguanshan has revealed that the origins of acumox can be traced back to periods before *The Inner Classic*. Consequently, our understanding and development of acumox theories can no longer be solely based on *The Inner Classic*. Moreover, modern acumox works, especially those from the Republic of China period, played an important role in the modernization of acumox and are an essential component in the development of acumox theory. Therefore, the literature coverage of *Selected Readings in Acumox Classics* spans from the silk books predating *The Inner Classic* to the Republic of China era, thus offering a more extensive coverage than typical Chinese acumox literature textbooks.

The specific arrangement instructions for *Selected Readings in Acumox Classics* are as follows:

1. The scope of acumox literature includes the key texts from the Qin and Han dynasties through to the Republic of China period. This encompasses unearthed documents such as silk books from the Mawangdui tombs, and bamboo-slip books from the Zhangjiashan and Laoguanshan tombs, as well as transmitted texts such as *The Inner Classic*, *The Classic of Questioning*, and *The Systematic Classic of Acupuncture and Moxibustion*, etc.

2. Select the key concepts of acumox theory, classify and compile significant acumox texts from the aforementioned works, and organize them chronologically from ancient times to the present based on their historical development to create a coherent theme.

3. According to the framework of modern acumox, the book is divided into three chapters: Meridians and Acupoints, Acumox Techniques, and Acumox Therapeutics. Each chapter is further divided into several sections, with each section including a general introduction, a discussion of development, notes, and reflections. The original text quoted in the development section is presented in a different style, and

some of the small characters within the original text are additional annotations or notes inserted by the ancient scholars. Due to the varying connotations of conceptual terms, some chapters may not follow the aforementioned style, but the overall concept remains consistent.

4. The English translation of TCM terminology is not yet standardized. At the end of each section, a comparison table is provided, listing the Chinese terms, their pinyin transliterations, and common English translations for key terms that appear for the first time in that section. The title of the book, when first mentioned, follows the format "*English book title* (*Pinyin*, Chinese book title)", for example, "*Huangdi's Inner Classic* (*Huáng Dì Nèi Jīng,* 黄帝内经)". In subsequent references, unless otherwise specified, only the English title will be used. When citing a specific chapter, the format used is "*Chapter name* of *English book title* (*Pinyin*, Chinese book title · chapter name)", for example, "*Nine Needles and Twelve Yuan-Source Points* of *The Spiritual Pivot* (*Líng Shū · Jiǔ Zhēn Shí Èr Yuán,* 灵枢 · 九针十二原)".

5. For certain background knowledge related to Chinese culture, history, works, and characters included in the textbook, a "Knowledge Database" has been established. Different text styles are used to introduce them. Terms that appear for the first time and those mentioned later are formatted similarly to the book titles. If a specific person is the author of a particular work, he will be mentioned in the introduction of the work; if the person does not have a related work, he will be introduced in the section dedicated to individuals. After each section, there is a list that summarizes the knowledge points introduced for the first time in that section.

6. The textbook includes an index and a bibliography at the end.

Selected Readings in Acumox Classics aims to help acumox learners from various countries gain a deeper understanding of the development and evolution of acumox theory, particularly those aspects that are inconsistent with and cannot be adequately explained by modern acumox theory. This textbook can be utilized for various forms of international acumox education and is also suitable for bilingual acumox teaching for Chinese students. At the same time, for acumox practitioners who use English, this textbook serves as a reference work to explore the development of acumox.

Due to the limitations of the editors' expertise, shortcomings and errors in this book are inevitable. We hope that readers will provide valuable comments and suggestions to help advance and improve acumox literature. Contact information: wj2018@shutcm.edu.cn.

Wang Jing
January 2025

Contents

Chapter 1
Meridians and Acupoints

Guidance

Understand the characteristics or connotations of the conceptual terms discussed in this chapter across different periods.

Be familiar with the titles of works from various periods related to the conceptual terms in this chapter.

Learn about the acupuncture cultural relics unearthed from the Laoguanshan and Shuangbaoshan tombs.

Topic 1

Jing Luo (Meridians and Collaterals)

1. General knowledge of Jing Luo

Jing Luo refers to the system of meridians and collaterals. Generally, this system includes twelve meridians, eight extraordinary vessels, twelve meridian divergences, twelve meridian sinews, twelve cutaneous regions, and fifteen collaterals, as seen in Fig. 1−1.

(Interior) — Zang-fu organs

↑

Jing Luo
- 12 meridians
- 8 extraordinary vessels
- 12 meridian divergences
- 15 collaterals

↓

(Exterior)
- 12 meridian sinews
- 12 cutaneous regions

(all of the above:) The System of Meridians and Collaterals

Fig. 1−1 A brief table of the system of meridians and collaterals

Among the meridians and collaterals, the twelve meridians are the main trunk, which "pertain to the zang-fu organs internally and connect with the limbs and joints externally", thus linking the internal and external parts of the body. The twelve meridian divergences are important branches of the twelve meridians, located in the chest, abdomen, and head. They strengthen the connections between the exteriorly-interiorly related meridians and facilitate communication between the meridians and the zang-fu organs. The fifteen collaterals are external branches of the twelve meridians in the limbs and the anterior, posterior, and lateral trunk; they connect the exterior with the interior and pour qi and blood. The eight extraordinary vessels follow unique pathways to govern and connect meridians, regulating the excess and deficiency of qi and blood. Tendons, muscles, and skin are divided into twelve meridian sinews and twelve cutaneous regions based on the distribution of meridians and collaterals. The theory of the eight extraordinary vessels was not completely developed in the *Huangdi's Inner Classic* (*Huáng Dì Nèi Jīng,* 黄帝内经) ("*The Inner Classic*") and is not covered in this section. It will be introduced in Topic 3.

KNOWLEDGE DATABASE: LITERATURE

Huangdi's Inner Classic (*Huáng Dì Nèi Jīng*, 黄帝内经)

Huangdi's Inner Classic, is also called *The Yellow Emperor's Inner Classic*. It is important to note that "Yellow Emperor" is only the literal translation of "Huang Di (黄帝)". "Huang Di" was not an emperor, but actually the name of a leader of an ancient tribe in China, and "黄帝" can also refer to the name of the tribe itself.

This book is usually referred to simply as *The Inner Classic,* which in pinyin is *Nèi Jīng* and in Chinese characters is 内经.

The Inner Classic is a book on the basic theory of TCM, mostly focusing on acupuncture and moxibustion. This book has a complicated history, and is generally believed to have been compiled by a group of authors over an extended period of time, with its final form completed during the middle and late Western Han Dynasty. Now the book is divided into two parts: *The Spiritual Pivot* (*Líng Shū*, 灵枢) and *Basic Questions* (*Sù Wèn*, 素问), each consisting of 81 chapters, typically presented in a question-and-answer format.

Ling Shu is sometimes translated as *The Miraculous Pivot*, while *Su Wen* can be translated as *Plain Questions*. Some scholars now suggest *Elementary Questions* as an alternative translation.

2. The origins and development of Jing Luo

2.1 Mai, Jing and Luo

The theory of meridians and collaterals was meticulously recorded in *The Inner Classic* and *The Classic of Questioning* (*Nàn Jīng,* 难经). Since then, scholars have explored the formation and development of the theory of meridians and collaterals based on these two classics. In the 1970s, silk books of *The Classic of Moxibustion on Eleven Vessels on the Feet and Arms* (*Zú Bì Shí Yī Mài Jiǔ Jīng,* 足臂十一脉灸经) ("*Feet and Arms* version") and *The Classic of Moxibustion on Eleven Vessels of Yin and Yang* (*Yīn Yáng Shí Yī Mài Jiǔ Jīng,* 阴阳十一脉灸经) ("*Yin and Yang* version") were unearthed from the Mawangdui tombs of the Han Dynasty in Changsha, Hunan Province. These texts include details on the circulatory pathways, indications and moxibustion techniques for the 11 vessels of the human body. In the 1980s, a bamboo-slip book named *The Book of Vessels* (*Mài Shū*, 脉书) was discovered in a Han Dynasty tomb at Zhangjiashan, Jiangling City, Hubei Province, and some of its contents were largely consistent with those found in the *Yin and Yang* version. These unearthed documents play an important role in the analysis of the development of the meridians and collaterals.

KNOWLEDGE DATABASE: LITERATURE

The Classic of Questioning (*Nàn Jīng*, 难经)

The Classic of Questioning is traditionally attributed to Bian Que, whose real name is said to be Qin Yueren, though this attribution is questionable. The book is dated to the Eastern Han Dynasty. It is commonly believed that the 81 chapters in the book aim to clarify difficult issues in the *Nei Jing*. However, some scholars argue that certain issues or ideas may not originate from *Nei Jing* but from other sources.

The book is also known by several other names, such as *Huangdi* (*Yellow Emperor*)*'s Classic of Eighty-one Difficult Issues*, *The Classic of Eighty-one Difficult Issues*, or simply *The Classic of Difficult Issues*. The character "难" is polyphonic, pronounced both nán and nàn. When pronounced as nán, the character "难" means "difficult", whereas when pronounced as nàn, it means "questioning". According to the content of this book, where "难" is understood to mean "questioning", a more accurate translation for the book is *The Classic of Questioning*. The number 81 refers to the total number of chapters in the book, each of which contains one or two questions along with their answers.

KNOWLEDGE DATABASE: HISTORY

The Mawangdui Tombs of the Han Dynasty

The Mawangdui tombs of the Han Dynasty (马王堆汉墓), located in Changsha City, Hunan Province, China, are the burial site of the marquis of Dai, Li Cang, and his family, who lived during the early Western Han Dynasty. There're 3 tombs, numbered 1 through 3 in chronological order, containing the remains of Li Cang's wife, Li Cang himself, and Li Cang's son, respectively.

In tomb No. 1, an almost perfectly preserved body of Xin Zhui, also known as Lady Dai, was discovered. In tomb No. 3, dated to the 12th year of Emperor Wen (168 BCE), several silk manuscripts were excavated in 1973. These manuscripts include the previously mentioned medical texts, as well as others such as the *Methods of the Vessel* (*Mài Fǎ*, 脉法).

KNOWLEDGE DATABASE: CULTURE

Silk books, bamboo-slip books

Silk books, silk texts, or silk manuscripts (帛书), refer to works written on silk. They're usually discovered in ancient tombs in China.

Bamboo-slip books (简书) refer to works written on bamboo slips. Bamboo slips (简) and wooden slips (牍) were the primary writing materials before the advent of paper in ancient China. Bamboo-slip books are also found in ancient tombs.

KNOWLEDGE DATABASE: LITERATURE

The Classic of Moxibustion on Eleven Vessels on the Feet and Arms (*Zú Bì Shí Yī Mài Jiǔ Jīng*, 足臂十一脉灸经)

This refers to one of the silk books unearthed from the Mawangdui tombs of the Han Dynasty.

Dated back to the pre-Qin period, the book outlines circulatory pathways, indications, and moxibustion techniques for 11 vessels named after the foot or arm.

The Classic of Moxibustion on Eleven Vessels of Yin and Yang (*Yīn Yáng Shí Yī Mài Jiǔ Jīng*, 阴阳十一脉灸经)

This refers to one of the silk books unearthed from the Mawangdui tombs of the Han Dynasty.

Dated to the pre-Qin period, the book introduces circulatory pathways, indications, and moxibustion techniques for 11 vessels named yin or yang.

KNOWLEDGE DATABASE: HISTORY

The Zhangjiashan Tombs of the Han Dynasty

The Zhangjiashan tombs of the Han Dynasty (张家山汉墓) are located in Jiangling County, Hubei Province, China. Tomb number 247 belonged to a low-level official who was skilled in law, proficient in calculations, interested in medicine, and practised daoyin—a form of physical exercise. The occupant of this tomb died in the 2nd year of Empress Lyu's reign, which corresponds to 186 BCE or shortly thereafter.

In this tomb, more than 1,000 bamboo slips were excavated in 1983–1984, and they could be categorized into various books. One of these books is *The Book of Vessels*, the bamboo-slip book mentioned earlier.

KNOWLEDGE DATABASE: LITERATURE

The Book of Vessels (*Mài Shū*, 脉书)

This refers to one of the bamboo-slip books unearthed from the Zhangjiashan tombs of the Han, dated to the 2nd year of Empress Lyu's reign (186 BCE), discovered in Jiangling City, Hubei Province in 1984.

Dated to the pre-Qin period, the book consists of five sections, which some scholars considered to be medical texts. The sections or books don't have titles. Since three of the five sections correspond to different ancient versions of silk books from the Mawangdui tombs, they are typically referred to by the names of these silk books, such as *The Classic of Moxibustion on Eleven Vessels of Yin and Yang* (Version C) and *Methods of the Vessel* (Version B).

In the *Feet and Arms* version and the *Yin and Yang* version, all meridians are named using the character "Mai (vessel, 脉)" or another ancient Chinese character for "Mai" ("温"), such as "arm Taiyin vessel", "shoulder vessel", "tooth vessel", etc. In *The Inner Classic*, "vessel" is also used to name meridians, such as "the lung vessel of hand Taiyin". "Vessel", one of the five tissues categorized as "skin, muscle, vessel, tendon, bone", originally referred to blood vessel. It denotes "blood-containing and multi-branched lines travelling inside the body (血理分斜行体者)". The use of the character "脉" reflects that ancient understanding of blood vessels were closely linked to the development of meridian and collateral theories in traditional Chinese medicine.

The term "Jing (meridian)" and "Luo (collateral)" emerged later than "Mai (vessel)". In *The Inner Classic*, "Mai" is categorized into "Jing Mai (meridian vessel, meridian)", "Luo Mai (collateral vessel, collateral)" and "Sun Mai (minute vessel, minute collateral)" based on their varying sizes and depths. Meridians and collaterals can be further classified into "deficient meridian", "excessive meridian", "yin meridian", "yang meridian", "yin collateral", "yang collateral", "big collateral", "small collateral" and "superficial collateral", depending on the deficiency or excess of qi and blood and their different distribution of yin and yang.

2.2 Eleven vessels, twelve meridians and other meridian theories in the early stage

2.2.1 Eleven vessels and twelve meridians

The *Feet and Arms* version and the *Yin and Yang* version are works from the pre-Qin period, whereas *The Meridians* of *The Spiritual Pivot* (*Líng Shū · Jīng Mài*, 灵枢 · 经脉) was completed later. There's an intrinsic relationship among the meridian theories presented in these three books.

KNOWLEDGE DATABASE: HISTORY

The pre-Qin period

The pre-Qin (先秦) period refers to the time before the Qin Dynasty (221 BCE-206 BCE) in Chinese history.

In a broad sense, the period spans over 1,800 years and includes various ancient stages, namely the Xia

Dynasty, the Shang Dynasty, and the Zhou Dynasty (which can be further divided into the Western Zhou Dynasty and the Eastern Zhou Dynasty). During this time, the ancient Chinese developed a rich and significant civilization. In an even broader context, the pre-Qin period may also extend back to the Paleolithic Era.

In a narrower sense, the pre-Qin period specifically refers to the Spring and Autumn period and the Warring States period, spanning from 770 BCE, when the Eastern Zhou Dynasty began, to 221 BCE, when the Qin Dynasty was established.

The Qin Dynasty

The Qin Dynasty (秦朝、秦代), the first imperial dynasty in China, was established in 221 BCE and lasting until 206 BCE. Its founder, Ying Zheng (嬴政), is more commonly known by his title, Qin Shi Huang (秦始皇), which literally means "the First Emperor of the Qin".

KNOWLEDGE DATABASE: LITERATURE

The Meridians of The Spiritual Pivot (Líng Shū · Jīng Mài, 灵枢 · 经脉)

The 10th chapter of the *Ling Shu*. It primarily addresses the names, starting and ending points, routes, symptoms, signs, and therapeutic principles of the 12 regular meridians and 15 collaterals.

There are 11 vessels recorded in the *Feet and Arms* version, including six "foot" vessels in the lower limbs: foot Taiyang, foot Shaoyang, foot Yangming, foot Taiyin, foot Shaoyin and foot Jueyin. Additionally, there are five "arm" vessels: arm Taiyin, arm Shaoyin, arm Taiyang, arm Shaoyang, and arm Yangming.

In the *Yin and Yang* version, a total of 11 vessels are recorded: 6 yang vessels, which include the foot Ju(Tai)yang, foot Shaoyang, foot Yangming, shoulder vessel (similar to the arm Taiyang vessel), ear vessel (similar to the arm Shaoyang vessel), and tooth vessel (similar to the arm Yangming vessel); and 5 yin vessels, which include the foot Ju(Tai)yin, foot Jueyin, foot Shaoyin, arm Ju(Tai)yin, and arm Shaoyin.

In *The Meridians* of *The Spiritual Pivot*, 12 meridians are recorded: the lung meridian of hand Taiyin, the large intestine meridian of hand Yangming, the stomach meridian of foot Yangming, the spleen meridian of foot Taiyin, the heart meridian of hand Shaoyin, the small intestine meridian of hand Taiyang, the bladder meridian of foot Taiyang, the kidney meridian of foot Shaoyin, the pericardium meridian of hand Jueyin, the Sanjiao meridian of hand Shaoyang, the gallbladder meridian of foot Shaoyang, and the liver meridian of foot Jueyin.

It's generally believed that the *Feet and Arms* version was produced earlier than the *Yin and Yang* version. However, from the viewpoint of content, the *Feet and Arms* version offers a more detailed distribution of the 11 vessels compared with the *Yin and Yang* version, and it also includes additional branches. In addition, the vessels in the *Feet and Arms* version were named according to three yin and three yang categories, whereas the names in the *Yin and Yang* version are more primitive, such as "shoulder vessel", "ear vessel", and "tooth vessel". These differences indicate that the two books originated from different sources. However, there are commonalities between the 11 vessels recorded in both books, such as:

- The vessels generally run towards the center, starting from the hand (wrist) or foot (ankle) and running towards the chest, abdomen, or head along the four limbs. However, in the *Yin and Yang* version, the "shoulder vessel" and the foot Ju(Tai)yin vessel run from the head or abdomen towards the tips of the four limbs.
- The courses of the vessels are relatively simple: some are merely connecting lines between the starting point and the end point, with few branches. In the *Feet and Arms* version, only the foot Taiyang and foot Shaoyang vessels each have two branches.
- The courses of the vessels are generally distributed on the surface of the body, with only a few running into zang-fu organs. For example, in the *Feet and Arms* version, the arm Taiyin "reaches the heart" and the foot Shaoyin "goes out of the liver". In the *Yin and Yang* version, the arm Ju(Tai)yin meridian "goes into the heart", the foot Shaoyin "links to the kidney", and the foot Taiyin "covers the stomach".
- There're no established links among the vessels in general. However, in the *Feet and Arms* version, it is noted that only the foot Jueyin vessel "intersects with the Taiyin vessel after ascending for 8 cun".
- Regarding to the order of the vessels, in the *Feet and Arms* version, the "foot" vessels precede the "arm" vessels. In contrast, in the *Yin and Yang* version, the "yang" vessels come before the "yin" vessels.

In *The Meridians* of *The Spiritual Pivot*, the courses of meridians are more systematized by incorporating interior-exterior relations between meridians, based on the distinctions of "hand", "foot", "yin", "yang", and the characteristic of meridians "internally pertaining to the zang-fu organs and externally linking the limbs and joints". Compared with the 11-vessel system, the 12-meridian system in *The Meridians* of *The Spiritual Pivot* has the following characteristics:

- The courses of the meridians run either upstream or downstream.
- Meridians include both an internal part that connects to the zang-fu organs and an external part that distributes to the body surface. The nomenclature of meridians also incorporates the related zang-fu organs.
- There're interior-exterior relations between meridians.
- Meridians are listed according to the order of three yin and three yang circulations.

The inheritance and development relationships between the 11-vessel and 12-meridian theories are illustrated in Table 1-1. It should be clarified that in the table, the arm Taiyin in the *Feet and Arms* version and the arm Juyin in the *Yin and Yang* version can't be directly equated to the hand Taiyin meridian in *The Spiritual Pivot*. However, from a nomenclature perspective, there're definite inheritance and development relationships. In the 11-vessel system, the arm Taiyin and arm Jueyin are described as "reaching the heart" and "entering the heart", with symptoms including "heart pain, vexation in the heart, and sighing" or "severe pain of the heart". These descriptions show more similarities with the hand Jueyin meridian than with the hand Taiyin meridian. After a comprehensive analysis of the routes and symptoms of the two vessels in the silk books, it suggests that the missing vessel in the silk books should be either the later lung meridian of hand Taiyin or heart meridian of hand Shaoyin. Further analysis of the route of the arm Shaoyin in the silk books reveals that both the arm Tai(Ju)yin and arm Shaoyin vessels contain elements of the hand Jueyin meridian from later periods. That is to say, during the era of the silk books, the content of the three yin vessels of the hand were mixed, and they were not clearly classified until later periods.

It's possible that the shift from the 11-vessel theory to the 12-meridian theory was influenced by cultural factors. In the pre-Qin period, there was a concept of "Heaven 6 and Earth 5". For example, in *Records of Melody and Almanac* of *The History of the Former Han* (*Hàn Shū · Lǜ Lì Zhì*, 汉书·律历志), it is stated that "6 corresponds to Heaven and 5 corresponds to Earth, and these numbers are constant. Heaven has six qi, which can descend and produce five flavours... The number 11 summarizes the principles of Heaven and Earth". In the 11 vessels, there were 6 yang vessels and 5 yin vessels, reflecting these numbers. The concept of "Heaven 6 and Earth 5" is also evident in the 25 points in the yin meridians (5 times 5) and 36 points in the yang meridians (6 times 6), as well as in the five zang and six fu organs in the theory of zang-fu organs. Later, the concept of circulation emerged in meridian theory. The number 12, originating from the *Book of Changes* (*Yì Jīng*, 易经) and signifying circular movement, more accurately reflects this theory. As a result, the number of meridians was adjusted from 11 to 12.

KNOWLEDGE DATABASE: HISTORY

The Han Dynasty

The Han Dynasty (汉朝、汉代) was the second imperial dynasty of China, beginning in 206 BCE and ending in 220 CE. This dynasty is divided into two periods: the Western Han (or Former Han), which lasted from 206 BCE to 9 CE and the Eastern Han (or Latter Han), which spanned from 25 to 220.

The Han Dynasty is regarded as one of the greatest dynasties in Chinese history. The majority ethnic group in China refers to themselves as the "Han group" and the Chinese script is known as "Han characters".

Table 1-1 Relations between the 11-Vessel System and the 12-Meridian System

	Feet and Arms Version	Yin and Yang Version	The Meridians of The Spiritual Pivot
Name of Meridian	温 (Mai)	脉 (Mai)	经脉 (Jing Mai)
Meridian Names (listed in the order of the original text)	Foot Taiyang	(Foot) Juyang	Lung meridian of hand Taiyin
	Foot Shaoyang	(Foot) Shaoyang	Large intestine meridian of hand Yangming
	Foot Yangming	(Foot) Yangming	Stomach meridian of foot Yangming
	Foot Shaoyin	Shoulder	Spleen meridian of foot Taiyin
	Foot Taiyin	Ear	Heart meridian of hand Shaoyin
	Foot Jueyin	Tooth	Small intestine meridian of hand Taiyang
	Arm Taiyin	(Foot) Taiyin	Bladder meridian of foot Taiyang
	Arm Shaoyin	(Foot) Jueyin	Kidney meridian of foot Shaoyin
	Arm Taiyang	(Foot) Shaoyin	Heart master meridian of hand Jueyin pericardium
	Arm Shaoyang	Arm Juyin	Sanjiao meridian of hand Shaoyang
	Arm Yangming	Arm Shaoyin	Gallbladder meridian of foot Shaoyang
			Liver meridian of foot Jueyin
Number of Meridians	11	11	12

KNOWLEDGE DATABASE: LITERATURE

Records of Melody and Almanac of *The History of the Former Han* (*Hàn Shū · Lǜ Lì Zhì*, 汉书 · 律历志)

The History of the Former Han, also known as *Qián Hàn Shū* (前汉书) or the *Book of (the Former) Han* ((*Qián*) *Hàn Shū*-(前)汉书), is a historical work primarily compiled by Ban Gu (32–92) during the Eastern Han Dynasty. This history covers the Western Han Dynasty, from the reign of its first emperor, Emperor Gao, beginning in 206 BCE to the fall of Wang Mang of the Xin Dynasty in 23.

The *Records of Melody and Almanac* section introduces the theory of musical tones and almanac.

Book of Changes (*Yì Jīng*, 易经)

Book of Changes, or *I Ching*, also known as *Scripture of Change*, is regarded as the first of the five classics of Confucianism. Originally a book of divination, it later evolved into a work of both philosophy and divination due to the explanatory appendices from the Confucian school. The book can be traced back to as early as the late Shang Dynasty and the early Western Zhou Dynasty (the 11th century BCE) and was composed by a group of authors over time.

2.2.2 Other meridian theories in the early stage

In addition to the 11-vessel/12-meridian theory, there were other schools of thought existed in the early stage of meridians. One instance is the carved lacquerware depicting human meridians, which was unearthed in 1995 from Tomb No. 2, a wood coffin tomb dating to the Western Han Dynasty, located in Shuangbaoshan, Yongxing Town, Mianyang City, Sichuan Province. The wooden figure was painted with 10 meridians, which can be categorized as three yin meridians of the hand, three yang meridians of the hand, three yang meridians of the foot, and the governor vessel according to the meridian theory in *The Inner Classic*. Although there are similarities in circulation with the 11/12 meridian system, there're significant differences. The meridian system depicted on the wooden figure for acupuncture use is an independent system.

KNOWLEDGE DATABASE: HISTORY

The Shuangbaoshan tombs of the Han Dynasty

The Shuangbaoshan tombs of the Han Dynasty (双包山汉墓) are located in Yongxing town, Mianyang city, Sichuan province, China. Among these tombs, Tomb No. 2 is believed to have been occupied by a chief executive of the local authority, possibly a descendant of the high nobility of the state of Chu. The tomb dates to the year before the fifth year of Yuan Shou (118 BCE) during the reign of Emperor Wu, the 7th emperor of the Western Han Dynasty. A lacquered figure of meridians was unearthed from this tomb.

In 2013, a lacquered figure depicting meridian points was unearthed in Laoguanshan, Tianhui town, Chengdu city, Sichuan Province. The figure features 22 red, thick lines on both sides of the body, which are bilaterally symmetrical and vertically distributed. Among the 11 red lines on each side, there're 5 on the front, 4 on the back, and 2 on the side. While 9 of these lines have running courses similar to the three yang meridians of the hand, three yang meridians of the foot, and three yin meridians of the foot as recorded in *The Meridians* of *The Spiritual Pivot*, the 2 red lines on the medial side of the upper limbs are different from any of the three yin meridians of the hand recorded in the same text. Besides, there're 29 white, thin lines carved in intaglio on the lacquered model, including 3 horizontal lines encircling the body and 26 vertical lines. Among the horizontal lines, the one at the level of the lower ribs is similar to the belt vessel described in *The 28th Issue* of *The Classic of Questioning* (*Nàn Jīng · Èr Shí Bā Nàn*, 难经 · 二十八难). Of the 26 vertical lines, 11 are on the front and 15 on the back and sides. The anterior middle line closely resembles the conception vessel mentioned in *The 28th Issue* of *The Classic of Questioning.* The remaining 25 vertical lines are all on the sides of the body, with most of them being bilaterally symmetrical. Some of the vertical white lines overlap with the red lines, and some also exhibit characteristics of the meridian courses recorded in *The Meridians* of *The Spiritual Pivot*. Certain sections resemble those of the three yin meridians of the hand, the three yang meridians of the hand, the three yin meridians of the foot, the foot Yangming meridian, and the foot Taiyang meridian.

In addition to the lacquered figure of meridian points, *Part 2* of *The Book of Vessels* (*Mài Shū · Xià Jīng*, 脉书 · 下经) was also unearthed from this Han tomb in Tianhui town. *Part 2* of *The Book of Vessels* is currently the earliest known written literature recording the meridian courses and symptoms of "the vessel of the heart master" and the "twelve regular meridians". Its meridian course direction is consistent with that in the *Feet and Arms* version, which is running in a single direction towards the center without showing the trends or characteristics of the circulation of the twelve meridians. However, there're 3 single branches: "foot Da(Tai)yang vessel", "foot Yangming vessel", and "foot Da(Tai)yin vessel" which share names with the regular meridians. The book also records the 9 extra vessels, such as "the Jianbiezan vessel", which are significantly different from those twelve vessels previously mentioned in *Part 2* of *The Book of Vessels*. Therefore, the contents of "the Jianbiezan vessel" is likely older than the twelve vessels, or even the *Feet and Arms* version and the *Yin and Yang* version. This suggests that there were multiple systems of meridians and collaterals at that time. These contents may reveal the early development of the meridian theory and are crucial for exploring of nature and origins of meridian concepts.

KNOWLEDGE DATABASE: HISTORY

The Laoguanshan (Tianhui) tombs of the Han Dynasty

The Laoguanshan tombs of the Han Dynasty (老官山汉墓), also known as the Tianhui tombs of the Han

Dynasty (天回汉墓), refers to the 4 tombs located in Tianhui town, Chengdu city, Sichuang province, China. Tomb No. 3 dates back to the reign of Emperor Jing (157 BCE–141 BCE) and Emperor Wu (141 BCE–87 BCE) of the Western Han Dynasty.

In 2012–2013, a lacquered figure of meridian points and several medical texts written on bamboo slips were excavated from Tomb No. 3.

KNOWLEDGE DATABASE: LITERATURE

The 28th Issue of *The Classic of Questioning* (*Nàn Jīng · Èr Shí Bā Nàn,* 难经·二十八难): This is the 28th issue of *The Classic of Questioning*. It explains the courses of the eight extraordinary vessels.

KNOWLEDGE DATABASE: LITERATURE

***Part 2* of *The Book of Vessels* (*Mài Shū · Xià Jīng*, 脉书 · 下经)**

This refers to a section of the bamboo slips unearthed from Tomb No. 3 of the Tianhui tombs of the Han Dynasty. This section was once divided into and named as 4 separate books. In earlier journals, it might be referred to by different names depending on the topic discussed.

The book contains 258 bamboo slips, mainly focusing on meridians and diseases. The 12-vessel theory, rather than 11-vessel theory, is already evident in this book.

2.3 Fifteen collaterals and the collaterals

In the classic literature on meridians and collaterals from *The Meridians* of *The Spiritual Pivot*, in addition to the 12 meridians, there are 15 collaterals. These include the collaterals of the three yin and three yang of the hand and foot, as well as the collaterals of the conception vessel, the governor vessel, and the major collateral of the spleen. In the original text, except for the major collateral of the spleen, all other 14 collaterals were referred to as "Bie (branch, 别)". Although 15 collaterals were also mentioned in *The Classic of Questioning*, the collaterals of the conception vessel and governor vessel are replaced by the yang collateral and yin collateral.

In addition to the collateral names mentioned above, *The Inner Classic* also describes zang-fu collaterals with properties similar to the "major collateral of the spleen". For instance, "the major collateral of the stomach is named Xu Li". However, both *The Inner Classic* and *The Classic of Questioning* list 15 collaterals, which may be related to the number "27". In *Nine Needles and Twelve Yuan-Source Points* of *The Spiritual Pivot* (*Líng Shū · Jiǔ Zhēn Shí Èr Yuán,* 灵枢·九针十二原), it is stated by "there're 12 meridians and 15 collaterals, totaling 27 qi". Yang Shangshan interpreted the number 27 as "3 times 9", which means "nine stars in the sky, nine districts on the earth, and nine orifices in the human body". This reflects the concept that "humans are an integral part of nature".

KNOWLEDGE DATABASE: LITERATURE

Nine Needles and Twelve Yuan-Source Points of *The Spiritual Pivot* (*Líng Shū · Jiǔ Zhēn Shí Èr Yuán*, 灵枢·九针十二原): The first chapter of the *Ling Shu*. It mainly introduces the nine needles, the 12 Yuan-source points, needling techniques for reinforcing and reducing, and various therapeutic principles.

In current textbooks, when introducing the Jing Luo system, it is noted that it consists of meridians and collaterals, typically mentioning only 15 collaterals as part of the Jing Luo system. However, in *The Inner Classic*, in addition to the 15 collaterals, there're also other collaterals, such as "the major collateral of the stomach" and minute collateral, which are also referred to as minute Mai. For example, in *The Length of Meridians* of *The Spiritual Pivot* (*Líng Shū · Mài Dù*, 灵枢·脉度), it is stated that "the Jing Mai is in the interior, their deviated routes are called Luo, and the branches of Luo are called Sun (minute)". So, the term "collateral" has a broad connotation. It may refer to the 15 collaterals, or the internal "Mai" connecting the zang-fu organs, such as "the major collateral of the stomach", or the minute branches of Jing Mai, including minute collaterals and blood collaterals, etc. In a word, the concepts of Jing and Luo are relative and can denote different structures depending on the context. Therefore, the "Luo" in ancient literature should not be automatically equated with the 15 collaterals.

KNOWLEDGE DATABASE: LITERATURE

The Length of Meridians of *The Spiritual Pivot* (*Líng Shū · Mài Dù*, 灵枢·脉度): The 17th chapter of the *Ling Shu*. It introduces the length of the meridians.

2.4 Twelve meridian divergences

The theory of the 12 meridian divergences is presented in *The Meridian Divergences* of *The Spiritual Pivot* (*Líng Shū · Jīng Bié*, 灵枢·经别). In this text, all the meridian divergences are referred to as the principal divergences (Zhèng, 正) of the three yin and three yang meridians of the hand and foot. At the beginning of the chapter, a question is posed: "The twelve meridians are involved in human life, disease occurrence, treatment, the origin of disease, the beginning of learning, and the goals of excellent doctors. This is the aspect that less skilled doctors may overlook, but experienced doctors will find challenging. Could you explain their separating, joining, resurfacing, and entering?" Qi Bo answered this question with an explanation of the 12 meridian divergences. From this, it is understood that the 12 meridian divergences are still considered part of the category of the 12 regular meridians.

KNOWLEDGE DATABASE: LITERATURE

The Meridian Divergences of *The Spiritual Pivot* (*Líng Shū · Jīng Bié*, 灵枢 · 经别): The 11th chapter of the *Ling Shu*. It mainly introduces the pathways of the 12 divergent meridians.

The meridian divergences branch off from the 12 regular meridians, a process known as "separating (or divergence)", followed by "entering" which means to enter the thoracic or abdominal cavities, "joining" which involves circulating with the corresponding interiorly-exteriorly related meridian divergences, and "resurfacing" which refers to emerging from the head and neck. The 12 meridian divergences form six pairs and circulate together to distribute through the chest, abdomen, and head. They can communicate within their pairs of interiorly-exteriorly related meridians, thereby strengthening their connections with the zang-fu organs.

The 12 divergent medians extend to areas that the 12 regular meridians don't reach, thereby broadening the indications for meridian points. For example, although the anus is not on the route of the bladder meridian of the foot Taiyang, points like Chengshan (BL57) on this meridian can still be used to treat hemorrhoids. This application of BL57 and similar points can be explained by the route of the foot Taiyang meridian divergence entering the anus, which enhances the theory of acupoint indications.

2.5 Twelve meridian sinews

In *The Meridian Sinews* of *The Spiritual Pivot* (*Líng Shū · Jīng Jīn*, 灵枢 · 经筋), the 12 meridian sinews are described and are categorized into the sinews of the three yin and three yang meridians of the hand and foot. According to *Elucidations of Script and Explications of Characters* (*Shuō Wén Jiě Zì*, 说文解字), "*Jin*" is defined as "muscles that can produce strength". In contrast, in *The Inner Classic*, the character "*Jin*" has various meanings, including tendons, muscles, superficial veins, and nerves. In *The Meridian Sinews*, "*Jīng Jīn*" primarily refers to muscles and tendons. These tendons and muscles form the 12 meridian sinews according to the distribution of the regular meridians. In *The Classified Classic* (*Lèi Jīng*, 类经) by Zhang Jiebin, a Ming Dynasty physician, the general distribution of the meridian sinews is summarized as follows: they all originate between the fingers and toes of the four limbs, become prominent at the supporting bones, connect at the elbows and wrists, link with joints and muscles, ascend to the neck and nape, and ultimately terminate at the head and face.

KNOWLEDGE DATABASE: LITERATURE

The Meridian Sinews of *The Spiritual Pivot* (*Líng Shū · Jīng Jīn*, 灵枢 · 经筋): The 13th chapter of the *Ling Shu*. It primarily focuses on the pathways of the 12 muscular meridians.

KNOWLEDGE DATABASE: LITERATURE

Elucidations of Script and Explications of Characters (*Shuō Wén Jiě Zì*, 说文解字)

Elucidations of Script and Explications of Characters is the first Chinese dictionary organized by components. It systematically analyzes the structure of Chinese characters and explores their origins. The book was compiled by Xu Shen, who lived during the Eastern Han Dynasty.

The Classified Classic (*Lèi Jīng*, 类经)

This book was compiled by Zhang Jiebin in 1624 during the Ming Dynasty. Zhang Jiebin, also known as Zhang Jingyue, used Jingyue as his literary name.

The author classified the contents of *The Inner Classic* into 12 categories in this work.

KNOWLEDGE DATABASE: CULTURE

Name, Courtesy name, Literary name

In traditional Chinese naming conventions, typical names consist of a family name (姓, xìng) followed by a given name (名, míng). The family name comes first, and the given name follows. Historically, besides the family and given names, individuals would also have a courtesy name (字, zì).

The courtesy name, or style name, is given during a coming-of-age ceremony, typically at the age of 20 for males and 15 for females. The courtesy name, usually bestowed by parents or respected elders, is often connected in meaning to the given name. After the coming-of-age ceremony, an individual is regarded as an adult, and others will use the courtesy name to show respect. However, superiors or elders will still address him by his given name. The person himself will use his given name to display modesty.

In addition to the given name and the courtesy name, some people also have a literary name (号, hào), which can be used by themselves and others to address them. The literary name is typically chosen by the person himself but can also be bestowed by others, such as seniors or even the emperor.

In history, for some famous and respected ones, neither their courtesy names nor their literary names were used in reference to them. Instead, people would use their official titles, their birthplace, the locations where they had served as officials, or notable features of their residences to address them.

Take Zhang Jiebin (张介宾) as an example: his family name is Zhang (张), his courtesy name is Huiqing (会卿), and his literary names include Jingyue (景岳) and Tong Yi Zi (通一子).

KNOWLEDGE DATABASE: HISTORY

The Ming Dynasty

The Ming Dynasty (明朝、明代) ruled China from the 14th century to the 17th century and is the second-to-last imperial dynasty in Chinese history.

The Meridian Sinews proposes a therapeutic principle for treating diseases of the meridian sinews: "Select the tenderness as the point". This principle is still commonly applied in the treatment of muscle and tendon issues today.

2.6 Twelve cutaneous regions

The cutaneous regions are the areas on the body's surface where the 12 regular meridians and their collaterals are distributed. The concept is primarily discussed in the *Discussion on the Cutaneous Regions* of *Basic Questions* (*Sù Wèn · Pí Bù Lùn*, 素问 · 皮部论). Since the nomenclature and diagnostic methods of the meridians with the same name are identical, the 12 cutaneous regions are also referred to as the 6-meridian cutaneous regions, resulting in only 6 distinct names (Table 1–2).

Table 1–2 6-meridian cutaneous regions

6-meridian Cutaneous Regions	Yangming	Shaoyang	Taiyang	Shaoyin	Xinzhu	Taiyin
Names	Hé Fēi (害蜚)	Shū Chí (枢持)	Guān Shū (关枢)	Shū Rú (枢儒)	Hé Jiān (害肩)	Guān Zhé (关蛰)

In the names of the 6-meridian cutaneous regions, "害 (He)" is interchangeable with "阖". "关 (Guan)", "阖 (He)" and "枢 (Shu)" refer to the latch, the leaf, and the pivot of a door, respectively. These terms not only denote specific areas on the body surface but also reflect the progression of the disease and changes in condition. Consequently, they provide insight into the analysis of 6-meridian diseases and mechanisms.

KNOWLEDGE DATABASE: LITERATURE

Discussion on the Cutaneous Regions of *Basic Questions* (*Sù Wèn · Pí Bù Lùn*, 素问 · 皮部论): The 56th chapter of the *Su Wen*. It mainly introduces the cutaneous regions.

The cutaneous regions can be used for diagnosis. Practical methods involve observing the superficial collaterals based on their distribution and color to determine the affected meridians and the nature of the disease. Specifically, "a predominance of blue indicates pain, black suggests bi syndrome, yellow-red points to heat, white signifies cold, and the presence of all five colors indicates a combination of cold and heat." Meanwhile, pathogenic evils can enter through the cutaneous regions: "When the evil is retained in the skin, it causes the muscular interstice to open. As a result, the evil can enter and invade the collaterals. Once the collaterals are filled, the evil will flow into the meridians, and when the meridians are full, it will get into the fu organs and zang organs. Therefore, the skin is divided into regions corresponding to the twelve meridians. If diseases in the regions are not cured, they can lead to more serious conditions."

In *Discussion on Inconsistent Needling* of *Basic Questions* (*Sù Wèn · Miù Cì Lùn*, 素问 · 缪刺论), the effects of the cutaneous regions in treatment are discussed. The text states, "... If there's pain without disease in the meridian, apply inconsistent needling techniques. Thus, locate the blood collaterals in the cutaneous region and treat them all." This principle has led to the development of techniques such as cutaneous needling and collateral pricking, which are based on the theory of cutaneous regions and inconsistent needling—a specific needling method for conditions in which the collaterals rather than the meridians are affected.

KNOWLEDGE DATABASE: LITERATURE

Discussion on Inconsistent Needling of *Basic Questions* (*Sù Wèn · Miù Cì Lùn*, 素问 · 缪刺论): The 63th chapter of the *Su Wen*. It introduces the technique of inconsistent needling—a specific needling method and addresses related issues.

3. Note

The ancient understanding of blood vessels evolved to the concept of "Mai (vessel)", which was later followed by the notion of "Jing Luo (meridians and collaterals)". In literature, the terms "blood vessels" and "meridians-collaterals" are sometimes used interchangeably, but they carry slightly different connotations. Generally, blood vessels often refer to perceptible vessels and the blood within them, while meridians-collaterals are more often used in functional descriptions such as connections and reflection within the body.

Jing Luo is an abbreviation for Jingmai (meridians) and Luomai (collaterals). The components of Jing Luo can vary across different treatises throughout history. Generally, Jing Luo consists of 12 regular meridians and 15 collaterals. Specifically, "Jing" typically refers to the 12 meridians, while "Luo" usually denotes the 15 collaterals. In some literature, the term "Jing Luo" is also used more broadly to refer to meridians.

Reflections

Compare the arm yin vessels and hand yin meridians across the 11 vessels of *Yin and Yang* version, the *Feet and Arms* version and the 12 meridians, and analyze the differences and similarities in their pathways and associated symptoms.

Terms and Synonyms

(1) History, culture and people

<table>
<tr><th>Term</th><th>Chinese</th><th>Explanations</th></tr>
<tr><td>The pre-Qin period</td><td>先 秦</td><td>The period before the Qin Dynasty (221 BCE–206 BCE)</td></tr>
<tr><td>The Qin Dynasty</td><td>秦 朝</td><td>The first imperial dynasty, 221 BCE–206 BCE</td></tr>
<tr><td>The Han Dynasty</td><td>汉 朝</td><td>The second imperial dynasty, 206 BCE–220 CE, being separated into two periods:
the Western Han (the Former Han) (206 BCE–9 CE);
the Eastern Han (the Latter Han) (25–220)</td></tr>
<tr><td>The Ming Dynasty</td><td>明 朝</td><td>The ruling dynasty from 1368–1644</td></tr>
<tr><td>Silk book</td><td>帛 书</td><td>Books copied on silk</td></tr>
<tr><td>Bamboo-slip book</td><td>简 书</td><td>Books copied on bamboo slips</td></tr>
<tr><td>The Mangwangdui tombs of the Han Dynasty</td><td>马王堆汉墓</td><td rowspan="4">Ancient tombs in China, dated to the Han Dynasty and unearthed after 1970s</td></tr>
<tr><td>The Zhangjiashan tombs of the Han Dynasty</td><td>张家山汉墓</td></tr>
<tr><td>The Shuangbaoshan tombs of the Han Dynasty</td><td>双包山汉墓</td></tr>
<tr><td>The Laoguanshan (Tianhui) tombs of the Han Dynasty</td><td>老官山汉墓
(天回汉墓)</td></tr>
<tr><td>Name</td><td>姓 名</td><td>A typical Chinese name consists of the family name and the given name</td></tr>
<tr><td>Courtesy name</td><td rowspan="2">字</td><td rowspan="2">The name one gets at his coming-of-age ceremony, usually given by parents or respected elders</td></tr>
<tr><td>Style name</td></tr>
<tr><td>Literary name</td><td>号</td><td>The name one makes for himself, or one gets from seniors usually</td></tr>
<tr><td>Huang Di</td><td rowspan="2">黄 帝</td><td rowspan="2">One of the Chinese mythological emperors</td></tr>
<tr><td>Yellow Emperor</td></tr>
</table>

(continued)

Term	Chinese	Explanations
Bian Que	扁鹊	An ancient Chinese physician who is also somewhat of a mythical figure; Qin Yueren was said to be Bian Que's real name
Qin Yueren	秦越人	
Xu Shen	许慎	The author of *Elucidations of Script and Explications of Characters*
Ban Gu	班固	The author of *The History of the Former Han*
Zhang Jiebin	张介宾	The author of *The Classified Classic*
Zhang Jingyue	张景岳	
Tong Yi Zi	通一子	

(2) Meridians and points

Term	Synonym	Chinese
Jing	• Meridian • Channel	经
Luo	Collateral	络
Mai	Vessel	脉
Bie	Collateral	别
Sun	Minute	孙
Zheng	Meridian divergence	正
Jin	• Sinew • Tendon	筋
Juyang	Taiyang	钜阳
Juyin	Taiyin	钜阴
Sanjiao	• Triple energizer • Three burners	三焦

(3) Book names

Term	Synonym	Chinese
The Classic of Moxibustion on Eleven Vessels on the Feet and Arms	*Zu Bi Shi Yi Mai Jiu Jing*	足臂十一脉灸经
The Classic of Moxibustion on Eleven Vessels of Yin and Yang	*Yin Yang Shi Yi Mai Jiu Jing*	阴阳十一脉灸经

(continued)

Term	Synonym	Chinese
Methods of the Vessel	*Mai Fa*	脉法
The Book of Vessels	*Mai Shu*	脉书
Huangdi's Inner Classic	• *The Yellow Emperor's Inner Classic* • *The Yellow Emperor's Inner Canon* • *Huang Di Nei Jing*	黄帝内经
	• *Inner Classic* • *Inner Canon* • *Nei Jing*	内经
The Spiritual Pivot	• *The Miraculous Pivot* • *Ling Shu*	灵枢
Basic Questions	• *Plain Questions* • *Elementary Questions* • *Su Wen*	素问
The Classic of Questioning	• *The Classic of Difficult Issues* • *Nan Jing*	难经
	Huangdi's Classic of Eighty-one Difficult Issues	黄帝八十一难经
The Classified Classic	*Lei Jing*	类经
Elucidations of Script and Explications of Characters	*Shuo Wen Jie Zi*	说文解字
	Shuo Wen	说文
Records of Melody and Almanac of the *History of the Former Han*	*Han Shu · Lü Li Zhi*	汉书·律历志
Book of Changes	• *Yi Jing* • *I Ching*	易经
	Zhou Yi	周易

(4) Chapters of *The Inner Classic*

The Spiritual Pivot

Term	Synonym	Chinese
Nine Needles and Twelve Yuan-Source Points	*Jiu Zhen Shi Er Yuan*	九针十二原
The Meridians	*Jing Mai*	经脉

(continued)

Term	Synonym	Chinese
The Meridian Divergences	*Jing Bie*	经 别
The Meridian Sinews	*Jing Jin*	经 筋
The Length of Meridians	*Mai Du*	脉 度

Basic Questions

Term	Synonym	Chinese
Discussion on the Cutaneous Regions	*Pi Bu Lun*	皮部论
Discussion on Inconsistent Needling	*Miu Ci Lun*	缪刺论

(5) Issues of *The Classic of Questioning*

Term	Pinyin & Chinese	Main Contents
The 28th Issue	*Er Shi Ba Nan*二十八难	Eight extraordinary vessels

Topic 2

12 Meridians and 14 Meridians

1. The ebb-flow of the 12 meridians and 14 meridians

1.1 The ebb-flow of the 12 meridians

The Meridians of *The Spiritual Pivot*: The hand Taiyin vessel of the lung... The hand Yangming vessel of the large intestine... The foot Yangming vessel of the stomach... The foot Taiyin vessel of the spleen...The hand Shaoyin vessel of the heart... The hand Taiyang vessel of the small intestine... The foot Taiyang vessel of the bladder... The foot Shaoyin vessel of the kidney... The hand Jueyin pericardium-collateral vessel of the heart master... The hand Shaoyang vessel of the triple energizer... The foot Shaoyang vessel of the gallbladder... The foot Jueyin vessel of the liver...

The Normal and the Adverse, The Fat and the Thin of *The Spiritual Pivot* (*Líng Shū · Nì Shùn Féi Shòu*, 灵枢 · 逆顺肥瘦): The three yin meridians of the hand run from the zang organs to the hands; the three yang meridians of the hand run from the hands to the head; the three yang meridians of the foot run from the head to the feet; and the three yin meridians of the foot run from the feet to the abdomen.

Yíng Qi of *The Spiritual Pivot* (*Líng Shū · Yíng Qì*, 灵枢 · 营气): Qi begins at the Taiyin and infuses into the hand Yangming. Then it flows upward to infuse into the foot Yangming. Proceeding downward, it travels to the dorsum of the foot and infuses into the big toe, merging with the Taiyin. From there, it ascends to the hip and infuses into the heart from the spleen. It flows along the Shaoyin, exits transversely from the armpit, runs downward along the arm, infuses into the little finger, and merges with the hand Taiyang. From this point, it redirects to flow over the armpit and then ascends to the medial side of the orbit and infuses into the inner canthus. Turning upward, it ascends to the vertex and then descends to the nape of the neck to merge with the foot Taiyang. Following the spine, it descends to the buttocks and flows into the tip of the little toe. From the sole, it infuses into the foot Shaoyin. It then ascends to infuse into the kidney. From the kidney, it infuses into the heart and externally spreads into the chest. Along the pericardium vessel, it emerges from the armpit and descends along the arm. From between the two tendons, it enters the palm, emerges at the tip of the middle finger, and returns to infuse into the tip of the fourth finger. Merging with the hand Shaoyang, it flows upward into the region between the breasts and spreads throughout the Sanjiao. From the Sanjiao, it infuses into the gallbladder, exits from the hypochondrium, and then infuses into the foot Shaoyang. It continues downward to the dorsum of the foot. From there, it infuses into the big toe, merges with the foot Jueyin, and ascends to the liver. From the liver, it infuses into the lung...

The theory of the twelve meridians was first introduced in *The Inner Classic* and is also known as the twelve vessels or twelve channels. In *The Meridians* of *The Spiritual Pivot*, the components of the twelve meridians and the path of each meridian are described, establishing the circulation pattern characterized by "adverse and normal running directions of vessels". This concept was further summarized in *The Normal and the Adverse, The Fat and the Thin* of *The Spiritual Pivot*, and later came to be known as "ebb-flow".

The twelve meridians regulate the circulation of qi and blood. Since the ying qi is contained within the vessels, its circulation follows the ebb-flow pattern of the twelve meridians. Typically, the meridians are organized according to their ebb-flow sequence rather than by the three yin and three yang categories. This sequence forms the structural basis for the continuous, circular flow of qi and blood within the human body. *Ying Qi* of *The Spiritual Pivot* provides a detailed description of this circular pathway.

KNOWLEDGE DATABASE: LITERATURE

The Normal and the Adverse, The Fat and the Thin of *The Spiritual Pivot* (*Líng Shū · Nì Shùn Féi Shòu*, 灵枢·逆顺肥瘦): The 38th chapter of the *Ling Shu*. It introduces needling techniques tailored to individuals with different physiological characteristics, illustrating their application in acupuncture. It also discusses the pathways of the 12 regular meridians.

Ying Qi of *The Spiritual Pivot* (*Líng Shū · Yíng Qì*, 灵枢·营气): The 16th chapter of the *Ling Shu*. It mainly focuses on the formation and circulation of ying qi, also known as nutrient qi.

1.2 The ebb-flow of 14 meridians

Ying Qi of *The Spiritual Pivot*: ...It ascends along the throat, enters the inner orifice of the nose, and runs deeper into the nasal cavity leading to the brain. One branch flows towards the forehead and vertex before descending to the nape of the neck. Along the spine, it travels to the sacrum, which is the pathway of the governor vessel. It circles around the genitalia, passes through the pubic hair, and enters the navel. From there, it travels upward along the interior of the abdomen to the supraclavicular fossa. It then descends, infuses into the lung, and remerges from the Taiyin.

Volume 9: Fifteen collaterals of *Grand Simplicity of "Huangdi's Inner Classic"* (*Huáng Dì Nèi Jīng Tài Sù · Juàn Jiǔ · Shí Wǔ Luò Mài*, 黄帝内经太素·卷九·十五络脉): The branch of the hand Taiyin is known as Lieque. The twelve regular meridians and the eight extraordinary vessels total twenty vessels, collectively referred to as meridians. Among these twenty vessels, there are twelve meridians, along with the governor vessel, the conception vessel, and the thoroughfare vessel, making up the fourteen meridians...

Explanatory Notes of *Elucidation on Fourteen Channels* (*Shí Sì Jīng Fā Huī · FánLlì*, 十四经发挥·凡例): The twelve meridians are listed in the order of their ebb and flow. Included are the two extraordinary vessels, the governor vessel and the conception vessel each with their own points. Together, they're referred to as the fourteen meridians.

Volume 6: *Illustrated Explanations of the Measurement of Point Location* of *The Complete Compendium of Ancient and Modern Medical Works* (*Gǔ Jīn Yī Tǒng Dà Quán · Juàn Liù · Qǔ Xué Chǐ Cùn Tú Shuō*, 古今医统大全·卷六·取穴尺寸图说): The length of the fourteen meridians: The six yang meridians of the hand... The six yin meridians of the hand... The six yang meridians of the foot... The six yin meridians of the foot... The governor vessel and the conception vessel... The two heel vessels... Together, the fourteen meridians measure sixteen *zhang* and two *chi* in length. This represents the great passageway of qi.

The concept of the fourteen meridians is thought to originate from *The Inner Classic*. After describing the circular pathway of the 12 meridians, such as "from the liver, it infuses into the lung", *Ying Qi* of *The Spiritual Pivot* further introduces the subsequent circulation pattern of the ying qi. The text "passes through the pubic hair, and enters the navel... travels upward along the interior of the abdomen" describes the course of the conception vessel in *Discussion on the Bone Holes* of *Basic Questions* (*Sù Wèn · Gǔ Kōng Lùn*, 素问·骨空论). That is to say, the circulation of ying qi starts from the hand Taiyin, travels through the twelve meridians, then the governor vessel and the conception vessel and finally returns to the hand Taiyin.

The term "fourteen meridians" first appeared in Yang Shangshan's *Grand Simplicity of "Huangdi's Inner Classic"*. The fourteen meridians referred to in this context include the twelve meridians as well as the three extraordinary vessels: the governor vessel, the conception vessel, and the thoroughfare vessel. As a result, the meaning of the term is relatively vague. Judging from Yang Shangshan's annotations on the thoroughfare vessel and the conception vessel in Volume 10 of *Grand Simplicity of "Huangdi's Inner Classic"*, Yang combined the conception vessel and the thoroughfare vessel into one. This synthesis was based on discussions of these two vessels in *The Inner Classic* and *The Classic of Questioning*, as well as references in other literature, such as *The Systematic Classic of Acupuncture and Moxibustion* (*Zhēn Jiǔ Jiǔ Yǐ Jīng*, 针灸甲乙经). This is why the term "fourteen meridians" was used.

Hua Shou's *Elucidation on Fourteen Channels* (*Shí Sì Jīng Fā Huī*, 十四经发挥) combines the conception vessel and the governor vessel with the twelve meridians to discuss the "fourteen meridians". This classification is based on the concept that both the conception vessel and the governor vessel have their own points, similar to the twelve regular meridians. Since Hua Shou's work was based on the lost text *Illustrated Point Location along Meridians from the Gold-Orchid Chamber* (*Jīn Lán Xún Jīng Qǔ Xué Tú Jiě*, 金兰循经取穴图解), the theory of the "fourteen meridians" may have existed even before Hua Shou's time.

In *The Complete Compendium of Ancient and Modern Medical Works*, Xu Chunfu quoted the text from *The Length of Meridians* of *The Spiritual Pivot* regarding the length of the twelve meridians, the governor vessel and the conception vessel, and the two heel vessels. He also used the term "fourteen meridians" or "fourteen vessels". This view was later adopted by *The Great Compendium of Acupuncture and Moxibustion* (*Zhēn Jiǔ Dà Chéng*, 针灸大成). However, the fourteen meridians discussed do not include the yin heel vessel and the yang heel vessel. As a result, in later generations, the concept of "fourteen meridians" generally adhered to Hua Shou's theory.

KNOWLEDGE DATABASE: LITERATURE

Grand Simplicity of "Huangdi's Inner Classic" (*Huáng Dì Nèi Jīng Tài Sù*, 黄帝内经太素)

Grand Simplicity of "Huangdi's Inner Classic", often abbreviated as *Tai Su* (太素), was compiled by Yang Shangshan. In this work, he classified the *Ling Shu* and *Su Wen* from the *Nei Jing* into various topics and provided annotations. This book, dating from the Tang Dynasty, was created to meet the emperor's requirements, similar to another of his works, *The Classified Bright Hall Theory of Huangdi's Inner Classic* (see below).

KNOWLEDGE DATABASE: HISTORY

The Tang Dynasty

The Tang Dynasty (唐朝、唐代) was the ruling dynasty from 618 to 907.

This period is considered a pinnacle of Chinese civilization. The Chinese take great pride in this era and sometimes use the term "Tang" to refer to themselves. For example, in many countries, there're districts known as Chinatown, where the population is predominantly of Chinese origin. The traditional Chinese translation of Chinatown is Tang Ren Jie, which means "street of Tang people".

KNOWLEDGE DATABASE: LITERATURE

Elucidation on Fourteen Channels (*Shí Sì Jīng Fā Huī*, 十四经发挥)

Elucidation on Fourteen Channels was written by Hua Shou in 1341 during the Yuan Dynasty, approximately 40 years after *Illustrated Point Location along Meridians from the Gold-Orchid Chamber* (see below). Hua Shou's book, which comprises three volumes, includes a note at the end of the second volume stating, "The previous two volumes are the same as *Illustrated Point Location along Meridians from the Gold-Orchid Chamber*". This indicates that Hua Shou copied the content from Hu Tai Bi Lie's book and added his own material to create a new work.

We can't judge Hua Shou or other historical figures by modern standards. In ancient times, despite advances in printing technology, the dissemination of knowledge was still challenging. Such coping practices actually contributed to the preservation and spread of knowledge as well as influence of the original authors, provided it was acknowledged in the new book.

The Complete Compendium of Ancient and Modern Medical Works (*Gǔ Jīn Yī Tǒng Dà Quán*, 古今医统大全)

The Complete Compendium of Ancient and Modern Medical Works is a comprehensive medical text written by Xu Chunfu in 1556 during the Ming Dynasty.

The book gathered medical materials from previous dynasties and was systematically classified and compiled into 100 volumes.

The Systematic Classic of Acupuncture and Moxibustion (*Zhēn Jiǔ Jiǎ Yǐ Jīng*, 针灸甲乙经)

The Systematic Classic of Acupuncture and Moxibustion, commonly referred to as *The Systematic Classic* for short, was compiled by Huangfu Mi in 282. The name "Huangfu Mi" features "Huangfu" as a compound or two-character surname, which is distinct from most Chinese surnames that typically have only one character.

This book gathered information related to acupuncture from *The Inner Classic*, *The Classic of Questioning* and *The Therapeutic Importance of Acupuncture Points from the Bright Hall* (see below), and established the theoretical system of acupuncture and moxibustion.

Illustrated Point Location along Meridians from the Gold-Orchid Chamber (*Jīn Lán Xún Jīng Qǔ Xué Tú Jiě*, 金兰循经取穴图解)

Illustrated Point Location along Meridians from the Gold-Orchid Chamber is a book written in 1303 during the Yuan Dynasty by a Mongolian author known as Hu Tai Bi Lie, or sometimes referred to as Hu Gong Tai. The book primarily covers the 14 meridians and their points, which include the 12 regular meridians, the governor vessel, and the conception vessel. All 14 meridians or vessels share a common characteristic: each has its own points. This book is the earliest to integrate the 12 regular meridians with the two of the eight extraordinary vessels.

Although the original book was lost, its content was preserved in *Elucidation on Fourteen Channels*.

The Great Compendium of Acupuncture and Moxibustion (*Zhēn Jiǔ Dà Chéng*, 针灸大成)

Yang Jizhou was a famous acupuncturist during the Ming Dynasty. He possessed a medical book from his family titled *Life-protecting Mysteries and Secrets of Acupuncture and Moxibustion* (*Wèi Shēng Zhēn Jiǔ Xuán Jī Mì Yào*, 卫生针灸玄机秘要), which served as the foundation for *The Great Compendium of Acupuncture and Moxibustion*.

The Great Compendium of Acupuncture and Moxibustion was written by Jin Xian, a medical official, and published in 1601 during the Ming Dynasty. It was originally compiled to honor Yang Jizhou's exceptional medical skills by one of his patients. Jin Xian expanded on Yang's family text by incorporating materials from other medical sources, making him the author of this compilation. However, Yang Jizhou is also considered as an author due to his significant contributions.

KNOWLEDGE DATABASE: LITERATURE

Discussion on the Bone Holes of *Basic Questions* (*Sù Wèn · Gǔ Kōng Lùn*, 素问·骨空论): The 60th chapter of the *Su Wen*. It mainly introduces point selection and needling techniques for various diseases. The term "bone hole" refers to the space between bones where acupoints are located.

Please note that the Chinese character "空" is typically pronounced as Kōng (the first tone), which means empty. However, in this title, it should be pronounced as Kǒng (the third tone), as it refers to a hole rather than "emptiness".

KNOWLEDGE DATABASE: CULTURE

Zhang (丈), Chi (尺)

Zhang (丈) and chi (尺) are both units of length, with 1 zhang equal to 10 chi.

There're also two other commonly used units of length: cun (寸) and fen (分). Specifically, 1 chi equals 10 cun, and 1 cun equals 10 fen.

The weights and measures were standardized when Emperor Qin Shi Huang unified China. However, in different periods and reigns, variations in measurement systems still existed. For example, while the names of the units mentioned above have remained the same, their actual lengths can differ.

2. The review of meridian point determination

2.1 *The Systematic Classic of Acupuncture and Moxibustion*

The Therapeutic Importance of Acupuncture Points from the Bright Hall (*Míng Táng Kǒng Xué Zhēn Jiǔ Zhì Yào*, 明堂孔穴针灸治要) is the earliest known acupoint text. Although it is now lost, its main contents are preserved in *The Systematic Classic of Acupuncture and Moxibustion*, authored by Huangfu Mi of the Jin Dynasty. In *The Systematic Classic of Acupuncture and Moxibustion*, the acupoints are organized according to the meridians on the limbs, starting from the tips, as well as by areas on the head, face, chest, and abdomen. This arrangement reflects the characteristics of centripetal single-direction approach in early meridian theories. Subsequently, texts such as *Formulas Worth a Thousand Gold Pieces* (*Qiān Jīn Fāng*, 千金方), *Classic of Nourishing Life with Acupuncture and Moxibustion* (*Zhēn Jiǔ Zī Shēng Jīng*, 针灸资生经) and some other generally adopted the same method.

KNOWLEDGE DATABASE: HISTORY

The Jin Dynasty

The Jin Dynasty (晋朝、晋代) ruled from 265 to 420. Like the Han Dynasty, it is divided into two periods: the Western Jin, which lasted from the beginning until 315, and the Eastern Jin, which spanned from 317 to the end of the dynasty.

Both dynasties share the name Jin, despite the brief interruption between them. At that time, people didn't distinguish between Western Jin and Eastern Jin; they simply referred to themselves as Jin. During the Jin Dynasty, the emperor's rule faltered but was later reestablished by descendants of the earlier emperors. They chose Nanjing, located east of the original capital Luoyang, as the new capital. Consequently, the terms "Western" and "Eastern" were used to differentiate between the two periods.

KNOWLEDGE DATABASE: LITERATURE

The Therapeutic Importance of Acupuncture Points from the Bright Hall (Míng Táng Kǒng Xué Zhēn Jiǔ Zhì Yào, 明堂孔穴针灸治要)

The Therapeutic Importance of Acupuncture Points from the Bright Hall is also referred to as *The Classic of Bright Hall Theory of Huangdi* (*Huáng Dì Míng Táng Jīng*, 黄帝明堂经), or simply *Ming Tang Jing*. It was completed around 80 to 106 during the Eastern Han Dynasty.

The author is unknown, but the book is regarded as the earliest known acupoint text. Although the original work has long been lost, its content is preserved in other ancient books like *The Systematic Classic of Acupuncture and Moxibustion.*

KNOWLEDGE DATABASE: CULTURE

Ming Tang, The bright hall

Ming tang (明堂) means "bright hall" or "bright mall". This term is quite famous in acupuncture. In ancient books, it often refers to the theory of meridians and acupuncture, especially when featured in the titles of medical books or figures.

Originally, the bright hall was a type of royal architecture where the emperor would conduct ceremonies or issue laws and decrees.

In *The Inner Classic*, it's said that Huang Di and Qi Bo discussed medical theories in the Ming Tang, or bright hall, and ultimately developed the theory of acupuncture. Huang Di later passed this theory on to his students in Ming Tang as well. Therefore, Ming Tang became an alternative term for acupuncture or meridian theory. However, it's important to note that Ming Tang can also refer to the nose or the body in some TCM texts.

KNOWLEDGE DATABASE: LITERATURE

Formulas Worth a Thousand Gold Pieces (Qiān Jīn Fāng, 千金方)

Important Formulas Worth a Thousand Gold Pieces for Emergency (Bèi Jí Qiān Jīn Yào Fāng, 备急千金要方)

Supplement to "Important Formulas Worth a Thousand Gold Pieces" (Qiān Jīn Yì Fāng, 千金翼方)

Formulas Worth a Thousand Gold Pieces can have two meanings. It can be an abbreviated title for *Important Formulas Worth a Thousand Gold Pieces for Emergency*. Alternatively, it can serve as a collective term for both *Important Formulas Worth a Thousand Gold Pieces for Emergency*, and *Supplement to "Important Formulas Worth a Thousand Gold Pieces"*.

Both books are comprehensive medical works in 30 volumes written by Sun Simiao, a scholar and doctor of the Tang Dynasty. He compiled *Important Formulas Worth a Thousand Gold Pieces for Emergency* around 652. Thirty years later, around 682, he compiled *Supplement to "Important Formulas Worth a Thousand Gold Pieces"* with the hope that this new work would elaborate the medical theories presented in his earlier book, much like wings to a bird. The Chinese term for "wing" is "Yi" (翼), which is literally translated as "supplement".

According to Sun Simiao's explanation, the phrase "a thousand gold pieces" in the book's title doesn't imply that the formula is worth 1000 gold pieces. Instead, it signifies that life is incredibly precious and more valuable than 1000 gold pieces.

Classic of Nourishing Life with Acupuncture and Moxibustion (Zhēn Jiǔ Zī Shēng Jīng, 针灸资生经)

Classic of Nourishing Life with Acupuncture and Moxibustion was written by Wang Zhizhong around 1180 during the Southern Song Dynasty. This book focuses on acupuncture and moxibustion.

In the *Book of Changes*, there's a Kun (坤) diagram, also known as Earth Diagram. Some commentaries on this diagram state, "Ultimate is the Kun principal, nourishing the life of all." As the second name suggests, this diagram represents the earth, which in TCM corresponds to the spleen and stomach. Wang Zhizhong titled his book "Nourishing Life", which is derived from the *Book of Changes*, and likely underscored his emphasis on the spleen and stomach. This perspective is evident throughout the book.

2.2 *The Classified Bright Hall Theory of Huangdi's Inner Classic (Huáng Dì Nèi Jīng Míng Táng Lèi Chéng,* 黄帝内经明堂类成)

During the Sui and Tang dynasties, under imperial order, Yang Shangshan compiled *The Classified Bright Hall Theory of Huangdi's Inner Classic*, which serves as an annotation to *The Therapeutic Importance of Acupuncture Points from the Bright Hall*. Only the first volume of this work has been preserved, including the author's preface and the content related to the hand Taiyin points. From the contents of the first volume, it's known that the original *The Classified Bright Hall Theory of Huangdi's Inner Classic* consisted of three volumes. However, in Yang Shangshan's version, there's one volume for each of the twelve meridians and one volume for the eight extraordinary vessels, totaling 13 volumes. In the first volume, the hand Taiyin points are arranged according to the ebb and flow of qi and blood within the meridian, establishing a precedent for point arrangement by meridian.

KNOWLEDGE DATABASE: HISTORY

The Sui Dynasty

The Sui Dynasty (隋朝、隋代) was the ruling dynasty from 581 to 618, lasting only 27 years. Despite its brief existence, it established the foundation for the succeeding Tang dynasty.

KNOWLEDGE DATABASE: LITERATURE

The Classified Bright Hall Theory of Huangdi's Inner Classic (Huáng Dì Nèi Jīng Míng Táng Lèi Chéng, 黄帝内经明堂类成)

The Classified Bright Hall Theory of Huangdi's Inner Classic, abbreviated as *Classified Bright Hall*, was written by Yang Shangshan during the Sui Dynasty. This book was intended to explain *Ming Tang Jing*.

According to the preface, *Ming Tang Jing* was composed of three volumes. Yang Shangshan's book classified the contents of *Ming Tang Jing* and organized the acupoints into different meridians. Thus, it's the first book to systemically arrange acupoints by meridians.

This book was also long lost, but at the end of the 19th century, its first volume was found in a temple in Japan. Historically, there were quite a few exchanges between China and Japan, particularly during the Tang Dynasty. During these exchanges, some Japanese monks traveled to China to learn and then returned to Japan, while some Chinese monks went to Japan, primarily to teach Buddhism and other knowledge, including medicine. A notable example is Jian Zhen, a Chinese monk who visited Japan six times and is highly respected in both countries. Since the remaining volume of *Classified Bright Hall* was found in a temple of Japan, it's likely that the book was brought to Japan by these monks.

2.3 *Arcane Essentials from the Imperial Library (Wài Tái Mì Yào, 外台秘要)*

In *Arcane Essentials from the Imperial Library*, written by Wang Tao during the Tang Dynasty, the 39th volume is titled "Moxibustion Techniques from the Bright Hall". This book organizes the acupoints along the meridians, attributing all points to the 12 meridians. Points on the conception vessel are attached to the part of the foot Shaoyin, while points on the governor vessel are attached to the part of the foot Taiyang. However, the order of the points does not always match the direction of qi and blood flow in the meridians.

KNOWLEDGE DATABASE: LITERATURE

Arcane Essentials from the Imperial Library (Wài Tái Mì Yào, 外台秘要)

Arcane Essentials from the Imperial Library, or Wai Tai for short, was compiled by Wang Tao. According to his preface, Wang Tao was an official who had long been in charge of the royal library. His interest in medicine arose from his own illness and that of his family. Thus, he took the chance to learn medicine in the library. When he was demoted to remote areas, it was his knowledge of medicine that enabled him to treat himself and recover from some serious illness. After this experience, he wrote this book.

However, Wang Tao may have encountered some unreliable acupuncturists, which led him to mistrust acupuncture. Hence, he only included moxibustion in this book, specifically in the 39th volume.

2.4 *Illustrated Classic of Acupoints on the Bronze Figure* (*Tóng Rén Shù Xué Zhēn Jiǔ Tú Jīng*, 铜人腧穴针灸图经)

During the Song Dynasty, under the emperor's order, Wang Weiyi compiled the *Illustrated Classic of Acupoints on the Bronze Figure*. This book features two types of point arrangements: One follows the system used in *The Systematic Classic of Acupuncture and Moxibustion*, while the other categorizes all points to 14 meridians and elaborates on the points according to their respective meridians. In the latter arrangement, the points of the 12 meridians begin at the tips of the extremities and progress towards the center. This method of arrangement was inherited from Yang Shangshan and also served as the basis for the *Illustrated Point Location along Meridians from the Gold-Orchid Chamber* written by Hu Tai Bi Lie (also called Hu Gong Tai) during the Yuan Dynasty.

KNOWLEDGE DATABASE: HISTORY

The Song Dynasty

The Song Dynasty (宋朝、宋代) ruled from 960 to 1279. It can be divided into two periods: the Northern Song, from its beginning until 1127, and the Southern Song, from 1127 to the end of the dynasty. The Southern Song period began when the empire lost control of northern China, had to relocate south, and established Lin'an, now part of Hangzhuo City in Zhejiang Province, as its capital.

The Song Dynasty was a prosperous era, vividly depicted in the famous painting *Along the River during the Qingming Festival* (清明上河图). However, from a knowledge perspective, the most significant development of this period was the enhancement of literature and knowledge due to the rapid expansion of woodblock printing, especially movable-type printing, which was invented in the 11th century.

KNOWLEDGE DATABASE: LITERATURE

Illustrated Classic of Acupoints on the Bronze Figure (*Tóng Rén Shù Xué Zhēn Jiǔ Tú Jīng*, 铜人腧穴针灸图经)

Illustrated Classic of Acupoints on the Bronze Figure was written by Wang Weiyi in 1026 during the Song Dynasty. Wang Weiyi, a medical official, compiled this work at the behest of the emperor.

In addition to the book, Wang Weiyi also cast two bronze figures to aid in the visual learning of acupoints. Although these original statues were lost over time, a bronze replica was made during the Ming Dynasty, and it's now housed in a museum in Russia.

2.5 *Elucidation on Fourteen Channels*

In Hua Shou's *Elucidation on Fourteen Channels*, the twelve meridians and their points are arranged according to the ebb-flow of qi and blood first, followed by the two vessels, the governor vessel and the conception vessel, and their points. From the perspective of acupoints, the points included in the fourteen meridians are more comprehensive. However, the positioning of the conception and governor vessels alongside the twelve meridians somewhat obscures the original ebb-flow concept of the twelve meridians, making the original meaning of the meridian theory more difficult to understand.

KNOWLEDGE DATABASE: HISTORY

The Yuan Dynasty

The Yuan Dynasty (元朝、元代) ruled China from 1271 to 1368. It followed the Song Dynasty and preceded the Ming Dynasty. This dynasty was established by the successor of Genghis Khan in China.

3. Note

From the single-direction flow to the center of the 11 vessels in the silk books to the ebb-flow of the twelve/fourteen meridians described in *The Meridians* of *The Spiritual Pivot*, the theory of meridians evolves from its original simple and straightforward form into a more complex and comprehensive system. Theoretically, the ebb and flow of qi and blood is central to the diagnosis and treatment of diseases in acupuncture and moxibustion. However, the qi and blood ebb-flow theory of the twelve or fourteen meridians can't explain all clinical phenomena, as it is neither the most comprehensive nor the only representative theory within the broader meridian system. On the contrary, it contradicts several other meridian theories in various aspects. For example, the theory that qi and blood become stronger from the extremities to the center, as represented by the five transport points (Jing-well, Xing-spring, Shu-stream, Jing-river, He-sea), and the theory of connections between the four limbs and the head, chest, and abdomen, represented by the branch-root and origin-terminal concepts, all present conflicting views. The theory of qi and blood ebb-flow in the twelve or fourteen meridians differs significantly from the initial concepts of meridian formation and provides limited practical guidance for acupuncture practice.

Reflections

What are the similarities and differences among the sequence of the 14 meridians, the point arrangement of these meridians, and the course of the ying qi?

Terms and Synonyms

(1) History, culture and people

Term	Chinese	Explanations
The Jin Dynasty	晋 朝	The ruling dynasty from 265 to 420 Being divided into two periods: the Western Jin: 265–315, and the Eastern Jin: 317–420
The Sui Dynasty	隋 朝	The ruling dynasty from 581 to 618
The Tang Dynasty	唐 朝	The ruling dynasty from 618 to 907
The Song Dynasty	宋 朝	The ruling dynasty from 960 to 1279. It can be divided into two periods: the Northern Song, 960–1127, and the Southern Song, 1127–1279
The Yuan Dynasty	元 朝	The ruling dynasty from 1271 to 1368
Zhang	丈	A unit of length, 1 zhang=10 chi
Chi	尺	A unit of length
Ming Tang	明 堂	A kind of architecture where the emperor held ceremony. In acupuncture, it usually refers to the theory of acupuncture of meridian
Huangfu Mi	皇甫谧	The author of *The Systematic Classic of Acupuncture and Moxibustion*
Yang Shangshan	杨上善	The author of *The Classified Bright Hall Theory of Huangdi's Inner Classic* and *Grand Simplicity of "Huangdi's Inner Classic"*
Sun Simiao	孙思邈	The author of *Formulas Worth a Thousand Gold Pieces*
Wang Tao	王 焘	The author of *Arcane Essentials from the Imperial Library*
Wang Weiyi	王惟一	The author of *Illustrated Classic of Acupoints on the Bronze Figure*
Wang Zhizhong	王执中	The author of *Classic of Nourishing Life with Acupuncture and Moxibustion*
Hu Tai Bi Lie	忽泰必列	The author of *Illustrated Point Location along Meridians from the Gold-Orchid Chamber*
Hu Gong Tai	忽公泰	
Hua Shou	滑 寿	The author of *Elucidation on Fourteen Channels*
Xu Chunfu	徐春甫	The author of *The Complete Compendium of Ancient and Modern Medical Works*
Yang Jizhou	杨继洲	An acupuncturist in the Ming Dynasty, the author of *The Great Compendium of Acupuncture and Moxibustion*
Jin Xian	靳 贤	The actual compiler of *The Great Compendium of Acupuncture and Moxibustion*

(2) Meridians and points

Term	Synonym	Chinese
Ebb-flow	Flow, Liuzhu	流注
12 meridians	12 channels	• 十二经脉 • 十二经
14 meridians	14 channels	• 十四经脉 • 十四经
Point arrangement by region		• 分部排列 • 分区排列
Point arrangement by meridian		按经排列
Centripetal (Centrifugal)	Toward (from) the center	向(离)心
Five transport points	• Five-Shu points • Jing-Xing-Shu-Jing-He points	五输穴
Branch-root theory	• Biao-Ben theory • Biao-tip and ben-trunk theory	标本理论
Origin-terminal theory	• Gen-Jie theory • Gen-root and Jie-knot theory	根结理论

(3) Book names

Term	Synonym	Chinese
The Therapeutic Importance of Acupuncture Points from the Bright Hall	*Ming Tang Kong Xue Zhen Jiu Zhi Yao*	明堂孔穴针灸治要
	• *Huang Di Ming Tang Jing* • *The Classic of Bright Hall Theory of Huangdi* • *Ming Tang Jing*	黄帝明堂经
The Systematic Classic of Acupuncture and Moxibustion	*Zhen Jiu Jia Yi Jing*	针灸甲乙经
	• *The Systematic Classic* • *Jia Yi Jing*	甲乙经
The Classified Bright Hall Theory of Huangdi's Inner Classic	*Huang Di Nei Jing Ming Tang Lei Cheng*	黄帝内经明堂类成
	Ming Tang Lei Cheng	明堂类成
Grand Simplicity of "Huangdi's Inner Classic"	*Huang Di Nei Jing Tai Su*	黄帝内经太素
	Tai Su	太　素
Formulas Worth a Thousand Gold Pieces	*Qian Jin Fang*	千金方
	Qian Jin Yao Fang	千金要方

(continued)

Term	Synonym	Chinese
Important Formulas Worth a Thousand Gold Pieces for Emergency	*Bei Ji Qian Jin Yao Fang*	备急千金要方
	Qian Jin Yao Fang	千金要方
	Qian Jin Fang	千金方
Supplement to "Important Formulas Worth a Thousand Gold Pieces"	*Qian Jin Yi Fang*	千金翼方
Arcane Essentials from the Imperial Library	*Wai Tai Mi Yao*	外台秘要
	Wai Tai	外　台
Illustrated Classic of Acupoints on the Bronze Figure	*Tong Ren Shu Xue Zhen Jiu Tu Jing*	铜人腧穴针灸图经
Classic of Nourishing Life with Acupuncture and Moxibustion	*Zhen Jiu Zi Sheng Jin*	针灸资生经
Illustrated Point Location along Meridians from the Gold-Orchid Chamber	*Jin Lan Xun Jing Qu Xue Tu Jie*	金兰循经取穴图解
Elucidation on Fourteen Channels	*Shi Si Jing Fa Hui*	十四经发挥
The Complete Compendium of Ancient and Modern Medical Works	*Gu Jin Yi Tong Da Quan*	古今医统大全
Life-protecting Mysteries and Secrets of Acupuncture and Moxibustion	*Wei Sheng Zhen Jiu Xuan Ji Mi Yao*	卫生针灸玄机秘要
The Great Compendium of Acupuncture and Moxibustion	*Zhen Jiu Da Cheng*	针灸大成

(4) Chapters of *The Inner Classic*

The Spiritual Pivot

Term	Synonym	Chinese
Ying Qi	*Ying Qi*	营　气
The Normal and the Adverse, The Fat and the Thin	*Ni Shun Fei Shou*	逆顺肥瘦

Basic Questions

Term	Synonym	Chinese
Discussion on the Bone Holes	*Gu Kong Lun*	骨空论

Topic 3

The Eight Extraordinary Vessels

1. The general knowledge of eight extraordinary vessels

The "eight extraordinary vessels" refer to the eight vessels that are not included in the twelve regular meridians. These include the governor vessel, the conception vessel, the thoroughfare vessel, the belt vessel, the yin heel vessel, the yang heel vessel, the yin link vessel, and the yang link vessel.

The original Chinese character for "extraordinary" is "奇", which has two meanings. One meaning is "extraordinary", referring to the distinct nature of the eight vessels compared with the twelve regular meridians in terms of distribution and function. The other meaning is "odd", as in odd and even numbers, suggesting something single and not in pairs. However, since the eight extraordinary vessels are not always unpaired, as seen with the yin heel and yang heel vessels, the yin link and yang link vessels,"奇" is typically interpreted as "extraordinary".

2. The development of the eight extraordinary vessels

2.1 The vessels of governor, conception, and belt before *The Inner Classic*

There's no record of these vessels in either *The Classic of Moxibustion on Eleven Meridians on the Feet and Arms* or *The Classic of Moxibustion on Eleven Meridians of Yin and Yang* unearthed from the Mawangdui tombs of the Han Dynasty in Hunan province, or in *The Book of Vessels* discovered in the Zhangjiashan tombs of the Han Dynasty in Hubei province.

On the lacquered sculpture of human meridians unearthed from the Shuangbaoshan tomb of the Han Dynasty in Sichuan Province, there're 10 painted meridians. Among these, one meridian runs along the midline of the body, starting from the pubic area, passing through the coccyx, sacrum, waist, back, and neck, reaching the vertex, then passing over the forehead, reaching the nose, and terminating at the tip of the nose. This pathway closely resembles the governor vessel described in *The Classic of Questioning* and *The Systematic Classic of Acupuncture and Moxibustion.*

In the pre-Qin text *Domination of Life Preservation* on of *Zhuang Zi* (*Zhuāng Zǐ · Yǎng Shēng Zhǔ*, 庄子 · 养生主), it's stated that "With Du (督) as the Jing (经), the body can be protected, life can be preserved, parents can be cared for, and the natural lifespan can be enjoyed" . This phrase "With Du (督) as the Jing (经)" is typically interpreted in two ways. First, according to the context, "督" is interpreted as "middle" and "经" as "regular way" suggesting that the phrase means to adopt the middle way as the universe law. In another explanation, which involves the theory of meridians and collaterals, "督" refers to the governor (Du) vessel. This interpretation emphasizes the importance of the governor vessel in preserving life. The concept of "the governing vessel" first appears in *The Inner Classic*, which was completed after *Zhaung Zi*. Initially, the former explanation, which interpreted "督" as the "middle" and "经" as the "regular way," was commonly accepted, but the discovery of the lacquered sculpture of human meridians from the Shuangbaoshan tomb suggests that the governor vessel could be a definite concept during the time of Zhuang Zi. Therefore, the latter explanation, which emphasizes the role of the governor vessel in life preservation, is also plausible.

KNOWLEDGE DATABASE: LITERATURE

Zhuang Zi (*Zhuāng Zǐ*, 庄子)

Zhuang Zi is a book named after its author, Zhuang Zi, meaning "Master Zhuang". He lived during the Warring States Period and is considered one of the most significant philosophers of Daoism. His ideas have also had a profound impact on Chinese literature and aesthetics.

Zhuang Zi is one of the foundational philosophical works of Taoism and a masterpiece of literature written by Zhuang Zi and his later scholars during the middle and late Warring States Period (476 BCE–221 BCE). It's also known as *The Authentic Classic of Nan Hua* (*Nán Huá Zhēn Jīng*, 南华真经), or *The Classic of Nan Hua* (*Nán Huá Jīng*, 南华经), as Zhuang Zi was honored with the title of Nan Hua True Man (南华真人) after the Han Dynasty.

There are 33 chapters in *Zhuang Zi*. The first 7 are known as the "Inner Chapters" (Nèi Piān, 内篇), which are generally considered to be the authentic works of Zhuang Zi. *Domination of Life Preservation* (*Yǎng Shēng Zhǔ*, 养生主) is one of these "Inner Chapters".

In 2013, a lacquered figure depicting meridian points was unearthed from the Laoguanshan Han Tombs. This figure features a white line along the anterior midline, which closely matches the pathway of the conception vessel as recorded in *The Classic of Questioning*, and can be identified as the conception vessel. Additionally, there is a white loop line at the level of the hypochondria, whose route is similar to the distribution of the belt vessel described in in *The Classic of Questioning* and can be regarded as the belt vessel.

2.2 The eight vessels in *The Inner Classic*

Orthodox Interpretation of Historical Records (*Shǐ Jì Zhèng Yì*, 史记正义), written by Zhang Shoujie of the Tang Dynasty, contains a note stating: "*Basic Questions* mention that the eight extraordinary vessels flow smoothly, but sometimes there are irregular intervals, which is referred to as the knotted pulse". This can be found in *Volume 105: No. 45 Biography of Bian Que and Cang Gong* of *Historical Records* (*Shǐ Jì · Juàn 105 · Biǎn Què Cāng Gōng Liè Zhuàn Dì Sì Shí Wǔ*, 史记 · 卷一百五 · 扁鹊仓公列传第四十五). This text does not appear in the existing *Basic Questions*. If it were a lost article from *Basic Questions*, the term "eight extraordinary vessels" is mentioned as early as in *Basic Questions*. However, according to the extant content, the term "eight extraordinary vessels" is not found in *The Inner Classic*.

KNOWLEDGE DATABASE: LITERATURE

***Orthodox Interpretation of Historical Records* (*Shǐ Jì Zhèng Yì*, 史记正义)**

***Historical Records* (*Shǐ Jì*, 史记)**

Historical Records is the first of China's 24 dynastic histories. The book was written by the Chinese historian Sima Qian between 104 BCE and 91 BCE.

Orthodox Interpretation of Historical Records, an annotation of *Historical Records*, was authored by Zhang Shoujie during the Tang Dynasty and was originally published as a separate edition consisting of 30 volumes. In the early Song Dynasty, its content was intentionally divided and integrated into the relevant sections of *Historical Records*.

Volume 105: No. 45 Biography of Bian Que and Cang Gong of *Historical Records* (*Shǐ Jì · Juàn 105 · Biǎn Què Cāng Gōng Liè Zhuàn Dì Sì Shí Wǔ*, 史记 · 卷一百五 · 扁鹊仓公列传第四十五) introduces Bian Que and Cang Gong, two famous doctors in Chinese history.

2.2.1 The conception vessel

Discussion on Points of *The Spiritual Pivot* (*Líng Shū · Běn Shù*, 灵枢 · 本输): The conception vessel is located in the Que Peng (broken basin) and is referred to as Tian Tu.

The Meridians of *The Spiritual Pivot*: The branch of the conception vessel is named Wei Yi (tail shadow). It descends to Jiu Wei (turtledove tail) and disperses in the abdomen. When there is an excess condition, pain in the abdominal skin may be observed, while in deficiency conditions, itching can occur. These conditions can be addressed by treating the branch.

Five Notes and Five Flavours of *The Spiritual Pivot* (*Líng Shū · Wǔ Yīn Wǔ Wèi*, 灵枢·五音五味): Both the thoroughfare vessel and the conception vessel originate from the uterus. They ascend along the interior of the spine and are considered the sea of meridians and collaterals. The superficial and exterior parts of these vessels run their own course along the abdomen, meet at the pharynx and larynx, and then separate, forming a circle around the lips and mouth.

Discussion on the Bone Holes of *Basic Questions*: The conception vessel originates below Zhongji (CV3). It ascends to the edge of the pubic hair, travels up along the abdomen to Guanyuan (CV4), reaches the pharynx and larynx, then rise to the chin, and finally enters the eyes along the face.

Discussion on Ancient Methods of Preserving Natural Essence of *Basic Questions* (*Sù Wèn · Shàng Gǔ Tiān Zhēn Lùn*, 素问·上古天真论): ...When a woman reaches her 14th year, Tian Gui arrives. At this stage, the conception vessel is open, and the thoroughfare vessel is in excess, resulting in regular menstruation and the possibility of pregnancy...However, by her 49th year, the conception vessel becomes weak, the thoroughfare vessel is deficient, Tian Gui is depleted, and the passageway of the earth is no longer open. Consequently, this leads to physical changes and infertility.

Discussion on the Bone Holes of *Basic Questions*: The diseases of the conception vessel include seven types of hernia in men, abnormal vaginal discharge in women, and various abnormal masses.

The descriptions of the conception vessel in *Discussion on the Bone Holes* of *Basic Questions* and *Five Notes and Five Flavours* of *The Spiritual Pivot* are essentially similar. However, the latter text specifies that the thoroughfare vessel and the conception vessel share the same origin and internal branches, while their external branches run separately. Despite this separation, they converge at the pharynx and larynx. *Discussion on Points* of *The Spiritual Pivot* simply notes that Que Pen is the area where the conception vessel passes. *The Meridians* of *The Spiritual Pivot* discusses the collaterals and diseases related to the conception vessel.

Meanwhile, *Discussion on the Bone Holes* of *Basic Questions* suggests that the conception vessel plays a role in women's pregnancy. The diseases described in this text align with the pathway of the conception vessel outlined in the chapter.

KNOWLEDGE DATABASE: LITERATURE

Discussion on Points of *The Spiritual Pivot* (*Líng Shū · Běn Shù*, 灵枢·本输): The 2nd chapter of the

Ling Shu. It primarily introduces points located below the elbows and knees, such as the five transport points.

Five Notes and Five Flavours of *The Spiritual Pivot* (*Líng Shū · Wǔ Yīn Wǔ Wèi*, 灵枢 · 五音五味): The 65th chapter of the *Ling Shu*. This chapter explores the correspondence between different types of people and the five musical notes, as well as the relationships among the five flavours, five zang organs, five fruits, five colours, and so on.

Discussion on Ancient Methods of Preserving Natural Essence of *Basic Questions* (*Sù Wèn · Shàng Gǔ Tiān Zhēn Lùn*, 素问 · 上古天真论): The first chapter of the *Su Wen*. It primarily focuses on the significance of health preservation for disease prevention and longevity, detailing methods for maintaining health. It also introduces the physiological processes of growth, aging, and fertility, with particular emphasis on the importance of kidney qi.

2.2.2 The governor vessel

Discussion on Points of *The Spiritual Pivot*: The governor vessel is located at the center of the neck (nape) and is known as Fengfu (GV16).

The Meridians of *The Spiritual Pivot*: The liver meridian of the foot-Jueyin... intersects with the governor vessel at the vertex.

The Meridians of *The Spiritual Pivot*: The branch of the governor vessel, known as Chang Qiang, runs along both sides of the spine, ascends to the nape, and disperses on the head. At the level of the shoulder blades, a branch connects with the Taiyang meridian, enters, and continues along the spine. Excess in this branch can lead to a stiff backbone, while deficiency can cause heaviness of the head... The point where the branch originates is used for treatment.

Ying Qi of *The Spiritual Pivot*: The foot Jueyin... ascends along the throat, enters the nasopharynx, and terminates at the posterior nasal aperture. Its branch runs up to the forehead, travels along the vertex, and descends to the nape, then continues along the spine to the sacrum, which is part of the governor vessel. This vessel then connects with the genitals, ascends through the pubic hair and enters the navel, and then moves upward along the interior side of the abdomen to enter Que Pen...

Discussion on the Bone Holes of *Basic Questions*: The governor vessel originates in the lower abdomen and descends to the center of the pubic bone. In women, it enters and connects with the urethral orifice—the opening at the tip of the urethra. Its collaterals run along the genitals, converge at the perineum, and then proceed to the area posterior to the perineum. One branch curves around the buttocks to connect with the Shaoyin meridian and intersects with the collaterals of the Taiyang meridian. The Shaoyin meridian ascends to the posterior area of the medial side of the thigh, penetrates through the spine and connects with the kidney. Another branch originates from the inner canthus, alongside the Taiyang meridian, travels up to the forehead, and then reaches the vertex, where it enters and connects with the brain. It then exits, and a branch descends to the nape, runs along the inner side of the scapula, reaches the waist along both sides of the spine, then enters and runs along the spine to connect with the kidney. In men, it runs along the penis and descends to the perineum, similar to the pathway in women. A branch that ascends directly from the lower abdomen penetrates the center of the navel, continues upward to pass through the heart, and then enters the larynx. It then ascends to the cheek, circles around the lips, and moves up to connect with the central areas below the two eyes. The diseases associated with it include pain rushing up from the lower abdomen to the cardiac region and issues with urination and defecation. This condition is known as rushing hernia. In women, it may lead to infertility, difficult urination, hemorrhoids, urinary incontinence, and a dry throat.

Discussion on the Bone Holes of *Basic Questions*: Diseases of the governor vessel may include stiff spines and opisthotonos.

The Meridians of *The Spiritual Pivot* states that the liver meridian of foot Jueyin "intersects with the governor vessel at the vertex". The text also provides a description of the collaterals of the governor vessel.

Both *Ying Qi* of *The Spiritual Pivot* and *Discussion on the Bone Holes* of *Basic Questions* describe the route of the governor vessel. However, in the former, the route generally runs from the top to the bottom, while in the latter, it's relatively complex. It originates from the lower abdomen, circles around the private parts, and ascends along the spine and back, with a branch running from the forehead to the vertex, and then descending along the back. In *Discussion on Points* of *The Spiritual Pivot*, it's stated that the center of the nape is the area where the governor vessel passes.

The descriptions of the governor vessel in both *Ying Qi* of *The Spiritual Pivot* and *Discussion on the Bone Holes* of *Basic Questions* contain texts similar to the route of the concept vessel described in *Discussion on the Bone Holes* of *Basic Questions*. This suggests a close relationship between the conception vessel and the governor vessel, with the possibility that they share a common origin but were named separately at a later stage. Referring to the description that "both the thoroughfare vessel and the conception vessel originate from the uterus" in *Five Notes and Five Flavours* of *The Spiritual Pivot*, Wang Bing proposed the theory of "three branches from one origin" in his annotations of this chapter. He stated that "the conception vessel, the thoroughfare vessel, and the governor vessel are three branches from one origin; this is why, in *The Inner Classic*, the thoroughfare vessel is sometimes referred to as the governor vessel. How do we know this? In the extant *The Systematic Classic of*

Acupuncture and Moxibustion and the ancient *Illustrated Classic of Meridian Circulation* (*Jīng Mài Liú Zhù Tú Jīng Tú Jīng*, 经脉流注图经), the route of the conception vessel along the back is referred to as the governor vessel, while the branch ascending directly from the lower abdomen is named both the conception vessel and governor vessel. Thus, these terms are used to distinguish between the back and the abdomen, as well as between yin and yang". This suggests that "the conception vessel, the thoroughfare vessel and the governor vessel are the same entity under different names".

KNOWLEDGE DATABASE: PEOPLE

Wang Bing (王冰)

Wang Bing (王冰) (c. 710–c. 804?), also known by his literary names "Qi Xuan Zi (启玄子)" or "Qi Yuan Zi (启元子)", was a scholar of the mid-Tang Dynasty. According to his writings, he devoted himself to health preservation and developed an interest in medicine from a young age. He held *Basic Questions* in high regard and spent 12 years completing his annotations of this text. His annotated version of *Basic Questions* (**see Topic 12**) became a foundational work for later generations' research.

KNOWLEDGE DATABASE: LITERATURE

***Illustrated Classic of Meridian Circulation* (*Jīng Mài Liú Zhù Tú Jīng Tú Jīng*, 经脉流注图经)**

Illustrated Classic of Meridian Circulation is a name mentioned in the in-text notes of *Basic Questions* by Wang Bing. It may refer to the title of a lost book, a lost illustration, or even a general term for medical works related to meridians and their circulation.

2.2.3 The thoroughfare vessel

The Normal and the Adverse, The Fat and the Thin of *The Spiritual Pivot*: The thoroughfare vessel is the sea of the five zang-organs and six fu organs, sustaining them all. Its upper branch exits at the nasopharynx, then penetrates and pours essence into all the yang meridians. Its lower branch flows into the major collaterals of Shaoyin, emerges in the region of Qi Jie (Street of qi), traces the medial side of the thigh, and enters the popliteal fossa. From there, it courses through the deeper layers of the leg and descends to the area posterior to the medial malleolus, where it diverges. The lower branch accompanies the Shaoyin meridian and penetrates the three yin meridians; its anterior branch continues deeper and exits at the upper edge of the calcaneus. It then descends along the calcaneus and enters the big toe, where it penetrates all collaterals and warms the muscles.

Pulsating Points of *The Spiritual Pivot* (*Líng Shū · Dòng Shù*, 灵枢·动输): The thoroughfare vessel is the sea of the twelve regular meridians. It originates below the kidney alongside the major collaterals of Shaoyin, emerges in the region of Qi Jie, and then travels along the medial side of the thigh, entering the popliteal fossa obliquely. It then runs along the medial side of the leg alongside the Shaoyin meridian, descends to the area posterior to the medial malleolus, and enters the region beneath the foot. A branch travels obliquely to the ankle, emerges to connect the upper border of the calcaneus, and then enters the big toe, where it infuses all collaterals and warms the foot and leg.

Five Notes and Five Flavours of *The Spiritual Pivot*: Both the thoroughfare vessel and the conception vessel originate from the uterus, ascend along the interior of the spine, and serve as the sea of meridians and collaterals. Their superficial and exterior parts follow their own course along the abdomen, converge at the pharynx and larynx, and then diverge to form a circle around the lips and mouth.

Discussion on Sudden Pain of *Basic Questions* (*Sù Wèn · Jǔ Tòng Lùn*, 素问·举痛论): The thoroughfare vessel originates from Guanyuan (CV4) and ascends along the abdomen.

Discussion on the Bone Holes of *Basic Questions*: The thoroughfare vessel originates from the region of Qi Jie, ascends along both sides of the navel together with the Shaoyin meridian and disperses upon reaching the chest.

Discussion on the Seas of *The Spiritual Pivot* (*Líng Shū · Hǎi Lùn*, 灵枢·海论): If there is an excess in the sea of blood, one may experience a sensation of an enlarged body and a feeling of depression without other obvious symptoms. Conversely, if there is a deficiency in the sea of blood, one may feel shrunk and constricted without other obvious symptoms.

Five Notes and Five Flavours of *The Spiritual Pivot*: Eunuchs have their Zong Jin (convergent tendons) removed, which damages the thoroughfare vessel. Consequently, the blood that is discharged can't be recovered and becomes coagulated beneath the skin, preventing nourishment to the lips and mouth, and the absence of facial hair.... For those born as eunuchs...it is due to congenital insufficiency qi, which results in inadequate development conception and thoroughfare vessels and a failure in the formation of Zong Jin. Where there is only qi present and the blood is absent, the lips and mouth can't be nourished, and as a result, the moustache can't grow.

Discussion on the Bone Holes of *Basic Questions*: Diseases related to the thoroughfare vessel include reversed qi and convulsive pain of the abdomen.

There're 5 discussions on the thoroughfare vessel in *The Inner Classic*. Among these, the descriptions in the chapters *The Normal and the Adverse, The Fat and the Thin* and *Pulsating Points* are similar.

The only difference is that the chapter *The Normal and the Adverse, The Fat and the Thin*, includes an additional upward route compared with the latter. In *Basic Questions*, the thoroughfare vessel ascends in both *Discussion on Sudden Pain* and *Discussion on the Bone Holes*. In *Five Notes and Five Flavours* of *The Spiritual Pivot*, the thoroughfare vessel has an interior branch that "ascend along the interior of the spine" and an exterior branch that "follow their own course along the abdomen". According to the descriptions in *The Normal and the Adverse, The Fat and the Thin* and *Pulsating Points* in *The Spiritual Pivot* and *Discussion on the Bone Holes* of *Basic Questions*, the thoroughfare vessel is considered to be bilateral meridians. However, according to *Five Notes and Five Flavours* of *The Spiritual Pivot* and *Discussion on Sudden Pain* of *Basic Questions*, it may also be viewed as a single vessel running along the midline.

In *Discussion on the Seas* of *The Spiritual Pivot*, either the sea of blood or the sea of twelve meridians refers to the thoroughfare vessel. The diseases of the thoroughfare vessel mentioned in this chapter manifest as abnormal sensations. *Five Notes and Five Flavours* of *The Spiritual Pivot* highlights the relationship between the thoroughfare vessel and blood, and it may affect the growth of a moustache. Both perspectives differ from those presented in *Discussion on the Bone Holes* of *Basic Questions*.

In *The Origin of All Diseases* of *The Spiritual Pivot* (*Líng Shū · Bǎi Bìng Shǐ Shēng*, 灵枢 · 百病始生), there are descriptions of "accumulation" related to "the vessel of subsiding rushing", which include the manifestation of a "pulsating under the hand when pressing". When *Wei Qi* of *The Spiritual Pivot* (*Líng Shū · Wèi Qì*, 灵枢 · 卫气) introduces the theory of Qi Jie, it states that "qi in the abdomen stops at the points of the back, as well as the pulsating vessels of the thoroughfare vessel on both sides of the navel". This "pulsating" may suggest that the formation of the thoroughfare vessel is connected to the pulsation of the abdominal aorta.

KNOWLEDGE DATABASE: LITERATURE

Pulsating Points of *The Spiritual Pivot* (*Líng Shū · Dòng Shù*, 灵枢 · 动输): The 62nd chapter of *Ling Shu*. It discusses why among the twelve meridians, the points on the three meridians of hand Taiyin, foot Yangming, and foot Shaoyin continually pulsate, and their relationship to the distribution and infusion of general qi and blood.

Discussion on the Seas of *The Spiritual Pivot* (*Líng Shū · Hǎi Lùn*, 灵枢 · 海论): The 33rd chapter of *Ling Shu*. It primarily focuses on the four "seas" in the human body: the sea of water and grain (the stomach), the sea of blood (the thoroughfare vessel), the sea of qi (Danzhong), and the sea of marrow (the brain).

Discussion on Sudden Pain of *Basic Questions* (*Sù Wèn · Jǔ Tòng Lùn*, 素问 · 举痛论): The 39th chapter of *Su Wen*. It primarily covers the etiology, pathogenesis, and fundamental features of various types of pain.

The Origin of All Diseases of *The Spiritual Pivot* (*Líng Shū · Bǎi Bìng Shǐ Shēng*, 灵枢 · 百病始生): The

66th chapter of *Ling Shu*. It primarily focuses on the etiology of diseases, introduces the pathogenesis and pathological mechanisms. The chapter emphasizes the significance of internal factors in the development of diseases.

Wei Qi of *The Spiritual Pivot* (*Ling Shū · Wèi Qì*, 灵枢 · 卫气): The 56th chapter of *Ling Shu*. It discusses the physiological functions of ying qi and wei qi (also known as defensive qi). It also covers the branch-root theory and the theory of qi pathways (**see Topic 4**).

2.2.4 The belt vessel

The Divergent Meridians of *The Spiritual Pivot*: The divergent branch of the foot Shaoyin meridian intersects with the Taiyang meridian when it reaches the popliteal fossa. It then ascends to the kidney and connects with the belt vessel at the fourteenth vertebra.

Discussion on Atrophy of *Basic Questions* (*Sù Wèn · Wěi Lùn*, 素问 · 痿论): The meeting point of Zong Jin is in the region of Qi Jie, where the Yangming meridian plays a central role. All these meridians connect with the belt vessel and the governor vessel. Therefore, a deficiency in the Yangming meridian can lead to the weakening of Zong Jin and a failure to properly regulate the belt vessel, resulting in atrophy of the foot.

There's only a brief mention of the route of the belt vessel in *The Inner Classic*. From a comprehensive view of all chapters in *The Inner Classic*, it is evident that the belt vessel is located around the fourteenth vertebra and is closely related to the divergent meridian of the foot Shaoyang and the Yangming meridian.

Discussion on Atrophy of *Basic Questions* suggests that the "failure to properly regulate the belt vessel" may lead to foot atrophy.

In *Epilepsy and Mania* of *The Spiritual Pivot* (*Líng Shū · Diān Kuáng*, 灵枢 · 癫狂), it is stated, "If the mania is located in the vessel, sudden collapse... if the vessel is not full, moxibustion can be applied to the Taiyang on the neck, Daimai (the same name as the belt vessel), which is on the waist, with a distance of 3 cun between the waist and this point, and to all flesh and points on the limbs". Here, "Daimai" should be referring to the point sharing the same name with the belt vessel.

KNOWLEDGE DATABASE: LITERATURE

Discussion on Atrophy of *Basic Questions* (*Sù Wèn · Wěi Lùn*, 素问 · 痿论): The 44th chapter of the *Su*

Wen. It primarily discusses the etiology, pathogenesis, and therapeutic principles related to atrophy.

Epilepsy and Mania of *The Spiritual Pivot* (*Líng Shū · Diān Kuáng*, 灵枢·癫狂): The 22nd chapter of the *Ling Shu*. It focuses on epilepsy and mania, including their etiology, types, and treatment methods involving acupuncture and moxibustion.

2.2.5 The yin heel vessel and the yang heel vessel

The Length of Meridians of *The Spiritual Pivot*: The heel vessel is a branch of the Shaoyin meridian. It originates behind the navicular bone, ascends above the medial malleolus, and travels straight upward along the medial side of the thigh, entering the pubic region. It then continues upward along the interior of the chest, enters the superior aspect of Que Pen, and emerges at the anterior of Ren Ying. It enters the cheek, and connects to the inner canthus. After meeting with the Taiyang meridian and the yang heel vessel, it ascends. The return of the combined qi from the yin and yang heel vessels can help moisten the eyes. If the qi can't circulate properly, the eyes may be unable to close.

Diseases of Cold and Heat of *The Spiritual Pivot* (*Líng Shū · Hán Rè Bìng*, 灵枢·寒热病): The foot Taiyang has an eye connection that enters the brain through the nape and directly links to the base of the eye. Pain in the head and eyes can be treated by focusing on the area between the two tendons on the nape. The eye connection links to the yin and yang heel vessels after reaching the brain. When the yin and yang vessels meet, the yang qi moves inward while the yin qi moves outward. The yin qi and yang qi converge at the inner canthus; thus, when the yang qi is excessive, the eyes open, and when the yin qi is excessive, the eyes close.

Invasions of Evils of *The Spiritual Pivot* (*Líng Shū · Xié Kè*, 灵枢·邪客): When reversed qi invades the five zang organs and six fu organs, wei qi can only defend the exterior and move within the yang areas, but it can't enter the yin areas. As it moves within the yang areas, yang qi becomes excessive, leading to fullness in the yang heel vessel. Since the qi can't enter the yin areas, yin deficiency results, causing the eyes to be unable to close.

Discussion on the Great Confusion of *The Spiritual Pivot* (*Líng Shū · Dà Huò Lùn*, 灵枢·大惑论): Huang Di asked, "What kind of evil causes insomnia?" Qi Bo replied: "This condition occurs because wei qi cannot enter the yin areas and remains in the yang areas. When it stays in the yang areas, yang qi becomes excessive, leading to fullness in the yang heel vessel. The inability to enter the yin areas causes a deficiency in yin qi, which prevents the eyes from closing." Huang Di asked, "What kind of evil causes eye problems in which the eyes can't see?"

Qi Bo replied, "This occurs when wei qi remains in the yin areas and cannot move into the yang areas. Staying in the yin areas leads to an excess of yin qi, which results in an overfull of the yin heel vessel. The inability to enter the yang areas causes a deficiency in yang qi, causing the eyes to close."

The courses of the heel vessels described in *The Length of Meridians* of *The Spiritual Pivot* primarily refer to the path of the yin heel vessel. The yin heel vessel originates from the navicular bone and travels to the inner canthus, where it intersects with the foot Taiyang and the yang heel vessel.

The Length of Meridians of *The Spiritual Pivot* highlights the close relationship between the yin and yang heel vessels and the eyes. Meanwhile, *Diseases of Cold and Heat* of *The Spiritual Pivot* emphasizes that these vessels meet at the inner canthus and regulate the opening and closing of the eyes. Consequently, disorders of the heel vessels primarily manifest as abnormalities in eye opening and closing, just as discussed in *Invasions of Evils* and *Discussion on the Great Confusion* of *The Spiritual Pivot*.

Discussion on Inconsistent Needling of *Basic Questions* states that "Evil invading the yang heel vessel of the foot will cause eye pain, which begins at the inner canthus. Needle two points half a cun below the lateral malleolus respectively...". This indicates that an invasion of evil in the yang heel vessel can cause eye pain starting from the inner canthus. However, since the entire chapter of *Discussion on Inconsistent Needling* focuses on collaterals, "the yang heel vessel of the foot" mentioned here should be interpreted as one of the collaterals.

In *Discussion on the Cave of Qi* of *Basic Questions* (*Sù Wèn · Qì Xué Lùn*, 素问 · 气穴论) and *Discussion on the Mansion of Qi* of *Basic Questions* (*Sù Wèn · Qì Fǔ Lùn*, 素问 · 气府论), references are made to "four points of the yin heel and the yang heel" and "one for each of the yin heel and the yang heel", respectively. Additionally, in *Diseases of Heat* of *The Spiritual Pivot* (*Líng Shū · Rè Bìng*, 灵枢 · 热病), it is noted that for "redness and pain in the eyes starting from the inner canthus, use the yin heel" and for "retention of urine, use the yin heel and the area above the three hairs, and let out blood in the blood collaterals". These references to "heel" are names of specific acupoints.

KNOWLEDGE DATABASE: LITERATURE

Diseases of Cold and Heat of *The Spiritual Pivot* (*Líng Shū · Hán Rè Bìng*, 灵枢 · 寒热病): The 21st chapter of the *Ling Shu*. It mainly introduces the manifestations, treatment, and prognosis of cold and heat diseases affecting the skin, muscles, and bones, including conditions such as bone bi and heat bi.

Invasion of Evils of *The Spiritual Pivot* (*Líng Shū · Xié Kè*, 灵枢 · 邪客): The 71st chapter of *Ling Shu*.

The chapter begins by addressing issues arising from the invasion of evil forces, then discusses the circulation of ying qi, wei qi, and zong qi, as well as various needle manipulation.

Discussion on the Great Confusion of *The Spiritual Pivot* (*Líng Shū · Dà Huò Lùn*, 灵枢 · 大惑论): The 80th chapter of the *Ling Shu*. It addresses the causes of blurred vision and dizziness and explores the pathogenesis of issues like poor memory and rapid digestion.

Discussion on the Cave of Qi of *Basic Questions* (*Sù Wèn · Qì Xué Lùn*, 素问 · 气穴论): The 58th chapter of the *Su Wen*. It primarily discusses the distribution of 365 acupoints. The term "cave of qi" refers to these acupoints, as each point is considered a place where the meridian qi converges.

Discussion on the Mansion of Qi of *Basic Questions* (*Sù Wèn · Qì Fǔ Lùn*, 素问 · 气府论): The 59th chapter of the *Su Wen*. It explains the number and distribution of acupoints associated with the meridian qi of each channel. The term "Mansion" refers to the meeting place of this qi.

Diseases of Heat of *The Spiritual Pivot* (*Líng Shū · Rè Bìng*, 灵枢 · 热病): The 23rd chapter of the *Ling Shu*. It focuses on the manifestations, diagnosis, treatment, and prognosis of heat-related diseases.

2.2.6 The yin link vessel and the yang link vessel

Treating Lumbago with Acupuncture of *Basic Questions* (*Sù Wèn · Cì Yāo Tòng*, 素问 · 刺腰痛): To needle the yang link vessel, locate it on the lower part of the calf where it intersects with the Taiyang meridian, approximately one *chi* above the ground.

Treating Lumbago with Acupuncture of *Basic Questions*: To needle the vessel of Feiyang, locate it 5 *cun* above the medial malleolus, anterior to the Shaoyin meridian, where it intersects with the yin link.

In *The Inner Classic*, the yin and yang link vessels are only mentioned in the chapter *Treating Lumbago with Acupuncture* of *Basic Questions*. However, based on the entire chapter, the terms "the yin link" and "the yang link vessel" (阴维 and 阳维之脉 in character) should refer to the regions to be treated rather than vessels.

KNOWLEDGE DATABASE: LITERATURE

Treating Lumbago with Acupuncture of *Basic Questions* (*Sù Wèn · Cì Yāo Tòng*, 素问 · 刺腰痛): The 41st chapter of the *Su Wen*. It discusses lower back pain caused by various meridians and outlines corresponding acupuncture treatments.

2.3 The eight extraordinary vessels in *The Therapeutic Importance of Acupuncture Points from the Bright Hall*

The Therapeutic Importance of Acupuncture Points from the Bright Hall, also known as *The Classic of Bright Hall Theory of Huangdi*, is the earliest known specialized book on acupoints. It's generally believed to have been compiled between the end of the Western Han Dynasty and 106 of the Eastern Han Dynasty. Although the original text has been lost for a long time, its main contents are preserved in *The Systematic Classic of Acupuncture and Moxibustion* written by Huangfu Mi of the Jin Dynasty, including the acupoint theories in volume 3 and the treatment of diseases in volumes 7–12.

In the 3rd volume of *The Systematic Classic of Acupuncture and Moxibustion*, there're descriptions such as "Part 2: On the head, 8 points in total on the line 1 cun above the hairline directly above the nose, along the governor vessel and turning to Fengfu (GV16)", "Part 3: On the head, 10 points in total on the line 1.5 cun lateral to the governor vessel then turning to Yuzhen (BL9)", "Part 7: On the back, 11 points in total from the first vertebra going down along the governor vessel to the sacrum of the spine", "Part 14: On the chest, 7 points in total from Tiantu (CV22) going down along the conception vessel to Zhongting (CV16)", "Part 15: On the chest, 12 points in total from Shufu (KI27), which is 2 cun lateral to the conception vessel, going down to Bulang (KI22)", "Part 19: On the abdomen, 15 points in total from Jiuwei (CV15) going down along the conception vessel to Huiyin (CV1)", "Part 20: On the abdomen, 22 points in total from Youmen (KI21), which is 0.5 cun lateral to Juque (CV14), going down along the thoroughfare vessel to Henggu (KI11)", "Part 32: 20 points in total of the foot Shaoyin and the thigh, including the yin heel and the yin link", "Part 34: 28 points in total of the foot Shaoyang and the thigh, and four points of the yang link", and "Part 35: 34 points in total of the foot Taiyang and 6 points of the yang heel". From these descriptions, the routes of the conception vessel, the governor vessel, the thoroughfare vessel, the yin and yang link vessels, and the yin and yang heel vessels can be deduced.

In the third volume, there're also points related to the eight extraordinary vessels. For example, Shenting (GV24) is the intersection point of the governor vessel, the foot Taiyang, and the Yangming; Benshen (GB13) is the intersection point of the foot Shaoyang and the yang link; and Touwei (ST8) is another intersection point of the foot Shaoyang and the yang link. The five points Shangxing (GV23), Xinghui (GV22), Qianding (GV21), Houding (GV19), and Qiangjian (GV18) are associated with the qi of the governor vessel. Tiantu (CV22) is the intersection point of the yin link and the conception vessel. The six points Xuanji (CV21), Huaguai (CV20), Zigong (CV19), Yutang (CV18), Danzhong (CV17), and Zhongting (CV16) are influenced by the qi of the conception vessel. Additionally, a total of 11 points from Youmen (KI21) to Henggu (KI11) are the intersection points of the thoroughfare vessel and the foot Shaoyin. Weidao (GB28) is the intersection point of the foot Shaoyang and the belt vessel, Zhaohai (KI6) is derived from the yin heel, and Shenmai (BL62) is derived from the yang heel, among others.

The ancient *Bright Hall* materials preserved in *The Systematic Classic* indicate that by the time when *The Classic of Bright Hall* was completed, the point attribution for the eight extraordinary vessels was already well-defined. This clarity was achievable only when the routes of the eight extraordinary vessels were firmly determined. Therefore, the formulation and completion of the theory of the eight extraordinary vessels likely preceded the compilation of *The Therapeutic Importance of Acupuncture Points from the Bright Hall.*

2.4 The eight extraordinary vessels in *The Classic of Questioning*

The theory of the eight extraordinary vessels presented in *The Classic of Questioning* had a profound influence on later periods, becoming the standard for subsequent discussions on these vessels.

2.4.1 The names and characteristics of the eight extraordinary vessels

The 27th Issue of *The Classic of Questioning* (*Nàn Jīng · Èr Shí Qī Nàn*, 难经 · 二十七难): There're eight extraordinary vessels, which are not controlled by the twelve regular meridians. What does this mean?

The answer is: The eight extraordinary vessels include the yang link vessel, the yin link vessel, the yang heel vessel, the yin heel vessel, the thoroughfare vessel, the governor vessel, the conception vessel, and the belt vessel. These vessels are not controlled by meridians, which is why they are referred to as the eight extraordinary vessels.

It's commonly believed that the term "eight extraordinary vessels" was first appeared in *The Classic of Questioning*. According to *The Classic of Questioning*, the term "extraordinary" in "eight extraordinary vessels" refers to their unique characteristic of being "not controlled by meridians".

KNOWLEDGE DATABASE: LITERATURE

The 27th Issue of *The Classic of Questioning* (*Nàn Jīng · Èr Shí Qī Nàn*, 难经 · 二十七难): The 27th issue of *The Classic of Questioning*. It explains the meaning of the term "eight extraordinary vessels" and why these vessels are not controlled by the twelve meridians.

2.4.2 The distribution of the eight extraordinary vessels

The 28th Issue of *The Classic of Questioning*: The governor vessel originates from the lowest point, runs along the inside of the spine, ascends to Fengfu (GV16), and then enters and connects with the brain.

The conception vessel begins below Zhongji (CV3), ascends to the pubic hair, runs along the interior of the abdomen and passes through Guanyuan (CV4), ultimately reaching the larynx and pharynx.

The thoroughfare vessel originates from Qichong (ST30) and ascends along with the Yangming meridian on both sides of the navel, dispersing upon reaching the center of the chest.

The belt vessel starts from the hypochondrium and encircles the body.

The yang heel vessel begins at the heel, travels upward along the lateral malleolus, and enters Fengchi (GB20).

The yin heel vessel also originates from the heel and ascends along the medial malleolus, reaching the pharynx and larynx, where it connects with the thoroughfare vessel.

The yang link and yin link vessels connect and integrate the entire body. They have functions related to exudation and storage, but they do not facilitate the circulation into other meridians. Thus, the yang link vessel originates from the area where all yang converges, while the yin link vessel originates from the area where all yin converges.

The 26th Issue of *The Classic of Questioning* (*Nàn Jīng · Èr Shí Liù Nàn*, 难经·二十六难): There're twelve meridians and fifteen collaterals. What are the additional three collaterals?

The answer is as follows: There are the yang collateral, the yin collateral, and the major collateral of the spleen. The yang collateral is associated with the yang heel vessel, while the yin collateral is linked to the yin heel vessel. This explains why there're a total of 15 collaterals.

The courses of the eight extraordinary vessels described in *The Classic of Questioning* differ somewhat from those in *The Inner Classic*. The routes of the conception, governor, and thoroughfare vessels are presented in a simpler manner compared with *The Inner Classic*. Additionally, the routes of the belt vessel, the yang heel vessel, and the yin and yang link vessels have been supplemented with further details.

According to *The Classic of Questioning*, the governor vessel runs along the posterior from bottom to top, the conception vessel runs along the anterior from bottom to top, and the belt vessel encircles the body transversely. These three vessels are single. The thoroughfare vessel, the yang heel vessel, and yin heel vessel, ascend from the lower to the upper and are bilateral. The yin and yang link vessels function more like a network that spans the entire body. It should be noted that the belt vessel originates from the hypochondrium, with a hypochondrium on each side of the trunk, meaning there're actually two belt vessels. However, because it "encircles the body", these two vessels merge into one.

The explanation of the 15 collaterals in *The Classic of Questioning* differs from that in *The Meridians* of *The Spiritual Pivot*. In *the 26th Issue*, the collaterals of the yin heel and yang heel replace the collaterals of conception and governor vessels as described in *The Meridians*.

KNOWLEDGE DATABASE: LITERATURE

The 26th Issue of *The Classic of Questioning* (*Nàn Jīng · Èr Shí Liù Nàn,* 难经 · 二十六难): The 26th issue of *The Classic of Questioning*. It explains the 15 collaterals, which differs from that in *The Inner Classic*.

2.4.3 The symptoms of the eight extraordinary vessels and their treatment

The 29th Issue of *The Classic of Questioning* (*Nàn Jīng · Èr Shí Jiǔ Nàn,* 难经 · 二十九难): The yang link vessel connects the yang, and the yin link vessel connects the yin. If yin and yang fail to connect with each other, it can lead to mental depression and a lack of control over actions. Diseases of the yang link vessel manifest as fever and chills, while diseases of the yin link vessel present as cardiac pain. Diseases of the yin heel vessel are characterized by the loosening of the yang and the tension of the yin, whereas diseases of the yang link vessel are marked by the loosening of the yin and the tension of the yang. Disorders of the thoroughfare vessel include reversed qi and convulsive abdominal pain. Diseases of the governor vessel are associated with a stiff and cold spine. Diseases of the conception vessel include internal coagulation, which manifests as seven types of hernia in men and abdominal masses in women. Diseases of the belt vessel are characterized by abdominal fullness and a sensation of weakness in the waist, as if sitting in water. These conditions pertain to the eight extraordinary vessels.

The 28th Issue of *The Classic of Questioning*: When the eight extraordinary vessels are affected by pathogenic factors, leading to swelling and a sensation of heat due to the accumulation of these evils, treatment can be administered by puncturing of a bian-stone.

In *The Classic of Questioning*, the diseases affecting the conception, governor, and thoroughfare vessels are similar to those described in *The Inner Classic*. However, the diseases of the yin and yang heel vessels are distinctly different from those in *The Inner Classic*, which primarily focuses on the eyes. Additionally, the diseases of the belt vessel and the yin and yang link vessels are introduced for the first time in *The Classic of Questioning*.

KNOWLEDGE DATABASE: LITERATURE

The 29th Issue of *The Classic of Questioning* (*Nàn Jīng · Èr Shí Jiǔ Nàn*, 难经 · 二十九难): The 29th issue of *The Classic of Questioning*. It explains the symptoms associated with the eight extraordinary vessels.

2.4.4 The functions of the eight extraordinary vessels

The 28th Issue of *The Classic of Questioning*: The yang link and yin link vessels connect and integrate the entire body. They have functions related to exudation and storage, but they do not facilitate the circulation into other meridians.

The 28th Issue of *The Classic of Questioning*: It's just like the ditches and lakes designed by wise men. When the ditches are full, the water naturally flows into the deep lake, a process beyond the control of the wise men. Similarly, when the human meridians are full, qi and blood flow into the eight extraordinary vessels and do not circulate further; this process is also beyond the control of the twelve regular meridians.

The Classic of Questioning compares the twelve regular meridians to "ditches" and the eight extraordinary vessels to "deep lakes". The eight extraordinary vessels function like deep lakes, serving purposes such as exudation and storage, but they don't participate in the circulation of qi and blood.

The Meridians of *The Spiritual Pivot* states that "The liver meridian of the foot Jueyin... meets the governor vessel at the vertex; its branch descends to the interior of the cheek from the eye connection, encircles the lips; another branch departs from the liver, penetrates the diaphragm and ascends to pour into the lung". In *Ying Qi* of *The Spiritual Pivot*, it explains that the circulation of ying qi begins at the hand Taiyin, travels through the twelve regular meridians, then moves through the governor vessel and the conception vessel, and ultimately returns to the hand Taiyin. That is to say, in *The Inner Classic*, the conception vessel and governor vessel are involved in the circulation of qi and blood through the meridians and are integral to this process. However, in *The Classic of Questioning*, the conception vessel and governor vessel are no longer part of the pathway of the qi and blood circulation within the meridians, which is the most important difference between the theories of the eight extraordinary vessels in *The Inner Classic* and *The Classic of Questioning*.

2.5 The eight extraordinary meridians in *Consideration of the Eight Extraordinary Vessels* (*Qí Jīng Bā Mài Kǎo*, 奇经八脉考)

Consideration of the Eight Extraordinary Vessels was written by Li Shizhen during the Ming

Dynasty. Drawing on references from *The Inner Classic*, *The Classic of Questioning*, *The Pulse Classic* (*Mài Jīng*, 脉经), *The Systematic Classic of Acupuncture and Moxibustion*, and *Formulas Worth a Thousand Gold Pieces*, the book incorporates the insights of medical experts like Zhang Zhongjing and Li Dongyuan, and thus provides a comprehensive supplement on the etiology, pathogenesis, pulse diagnosis, treatment, and formulas related to the eight extraordinary vessels. Furthermore, the book integrates theories from Taoism and compares them with medical theories.

Consideration of the Eight Extraordinary Vessels summarizes the functions of the eight extraordinary vessels as follows: "The governor vessel... is the general regulator of all yang vessels, hence it's called the sea of yang vessels. The conception vessel is known as the sea of yin vessels. The thoroughfare vessel... acts as the conduit for all vessels, which is why it's called the sea of the twelve regular meridians. The belt vessel... generally controls all vessels. Thus, the yang link vessel controls the exterior of the entire body, while the yin link vessel governs the interior... The yang heel vessel regulates yang throughout the body, whereas the yin heel vessel regulates yin... The governor vessel manages the yang of the posterior, while the conception and thoroughfare vessels control the yin of the anterior...The belt vessel restricts all vessels transversely". These texts have significantly impacted subsequent research on the eight extraordinary vessels.

KNOWLEDGE DATABASE: LITERATURE

Consideration of the Eight Extraordinary Vessels (*Qí Jīng Bā Mài Kǎo*, 奇经八脉考)

Consideration of the Eight Extraordinary Vessels was compiled by Li Shizhen (c. 1518–1593) in 1577 during the Ming Dynasty. This book explores the circulation, major diseases, and acupoints associated with the eight extraordinary vessels.

The Pulse Classic (*Mài Jīng*, 脉经)

The Pulse Classic was written by Wang Shuhe during the Western Jin Dynasty in the 3rd century. It is the earliest surviving monograph on pulse theory in China.

KNOWLEDGE DATABASE: PEOPLE

Zhang Zhongjing (张仲景)

Zhang Ji, courtesy name Zhongjing, was a renowned physician in the late Eastern Han Dynasty and is celebrated as the "Sage of Medicine" by later generations. He extensively compiled medical prescriptions and authored the *Treatise on Cold Damage and Miscellaneous Diseases* (*Shāng Hán Zá Bìng Lùn*, 伤寒杂病论) (**see Topic 10**), which established the foundational principle of "treatment according to syndrome differentiation" in traditional Chinese medicine.

Li Dongyuan (李东垣)

Dongyuan was the literary name of Li Gao (1180–1251), which is more commonly known than his courtesy name, Mingzhi. Li Dongyuan was a physician during the Jin (Kin) Dynasty and is recognized as one of the "Four Great Masters of the Jin and Yuan dynasties". He's the founder of the "spleen and stomach theory" in T.C.M., emphasizing the crucial role of the spleen and stomach in the human body.

3. Note

The Inner Classic provides a detailed discussion on the circulation of the governor vessel, the conception vessel, and the thoroughfare vessel. While the texts complement each other, they also present some contradictions, reflecting the early development of the theory of the eight extraordinary vessels.

Reflections

Read and compare the descriptions of the circulation patterns of the governor vessel, the conception vessel, and the thoroughfare vessel in *The Inner Classic*, and create a schematic diagram illustrating the concept of "three branches from one origin".

Terms and Synonyms

(1) History, culture and people

<table>
<tr><th>Term</th><th>Chinese</th><th>Explanations</th></tr>
<tr><td>Zhuang Zi</td><td>庄　子</td><td rowspan="3">The author of Zhuang Zi</td></tr>
<tr><td>Zhuang Zhou</td><td>庄　周</td></tr>
<tr><td>Nan Hua True Man</td><td>南华真人</td></tr>
<tr><td>Sima Qian</td><td>司马迁</td><td>The author of Historical Records</td></tr>
<tr><td>Zhang Ji</td><td>张　机</td><td rowspan="2">The author of Treatise on Cold Damage and Miscellaneous Diseases</td></tr>
<tr><td>Zhang Zhongjing</td><td>张仲景</td></tr>
<tr><td>Wang Shuhe</td><td>王叔和</td><td>The author of The Pulse Classic</td></tr>
<tr><td>Zhang Shoujie</td><td>张守节</td><td>The author of Orthodox Interpretation of Historical Records</td></tr>
<tr><td>Wang Bing</td><td>王　冰</td><td rowspan="2">A scholar from the middle Tang Dynasty, famous for his annotations to Basic Questions</td></tr>
<tr><td>Qi Xuan Zi</td><td>启玄子</td></tr>
</table>

(continued)

Term	Chinese	Explanations
Qi Yuan Zi	启元子	A scholar from the middle Tang Dynasty, famous for his annotations to *Basic Questions*
Li Gao	李　杲	A doctor from the Jin (Kin) Dynasty
Li Mingzhi	李明之	
Li Dongyuan	李东垣	
Li Shizhen	李时珍	The author of *Consideration of the Eight Extraordinary Vessels*

(2) Meridians and points

Term	Synonym	Chinese
Eight Extraordinary Vessels	Eight extraordinary meridians	奇经八脉
Governor vessel	Du meridian	督　脉
Conception vessel	Ren meridian	任　脉
Thoroughfare vessel	Chong meridian	冲　脉
Belt vessel	Dai meridian	带　脉
Yang heel vessel	Yangqiao meridian	阳跷脉
Yin heel vessel	Yinqiao meridian	阴跷脉
Yang link vessel	Yangwei meridian	阳维脉
Yin link vessel	Yinwei meridian	阴维脉

(3) Book names

Term	Synonym	Chinese
The Pulse Classic	*Mai Jing*	脉　经
Illustrated Classic of Meridian Circulation	*Jing Mai Liu Zhu Tu Jing*	经脉流注图经
Consideration of the Eight Extraordinary Vessels	*Qi Jing Ba Mai Kao*	奇经八脉考

(continued)

Term	Synonym	Chinese
Zhuang Zi		庄 子
	• *The Authentic Classic of Nan Hua* • *Nan Hua Zhen Jing*	南华真经
	• *The Classic of Nan Hua* • *Nan Hua Jing*	南华经
Historical Records	*Shi Ji*	史 记
Orthodox Interpretation of Historical Records	*Shi Ji Zheng Yi*	史记正义

(4) Chapters of *The Inner Classic*

The Spiritual Pivot

Term	Synonym	Chinese
Discussion on Points	*Ben Shu*	本 输
Diseases of Cold and Heat	*Han Re Bing*	寒热病
Epilepsy and Mania	*Dian Kuang*	癫 狂
Diseases of Heat	*Re Bing*	热 病
Discussion on the Seas	*Hai Lun*	海 论
Wei Qi	*Wei Qi*	卫 气
Pulsating Points	*Dong Shu*	动 输
Five Notes and Five Flavours	*Wu Yin Wu Wei*	五音五味
The Origin of All Diseases	*Bai Bing Shi Sheng*	百病始生
Invasion of Evils	*Xie Ke*	邪 客
Discussion on the Great Confusion	*Da Huo Lun*	大惑论

Basic Questions

Term	Synonym	Chinese
Discussion on Ancient Methods of Preserving Natural Essence	*Shang Gu Tian Zhen Lun*	上古天真论
Discussion on Sudden Pain	*Ju Tong Lun*	举痛论

(continued)

Term	Synonym	Chinese
Treating Lumbago with Acupuncture	*Ci Yao Tong*	刺腰痛
Discussion on Atrophy	*Wei Lun*	痿 论
Discussion on the Cave of Qi	*Qi Xue Lun*	气穴论
Discussion on the Mansion of Qi	*Qi Fu Lun*	气府论

(5) Issues of *The Classic of Questioning*

Term	Pinyin & Chinese	Main Contents
The 26th Issue	*Er Shi Liu Nan* 二十六难	15 collaterals
The 27th Issue	*Er Shi Qi Nan* 二十七难	Eight extraordinary vessels
The 29th Issue	*Er Shi Jiu Nan* 二十九难	Eight extraordinary vessels

Topic 4

The Pattern of Meridian Point Arrangement

1. General knowledge of meridian point arrangement

In modern acupuncture textbooks, the acupoints of the twelve regular meridians are arranged according to the sequence of qi and blood flow through these meridians. Generally, the twelve regular meridians are listed according to the ebb-flow of qi and blood. Within each meridian, acupoints on the three hand yin meridians are arranged from the chest to the hand, those on the three hand yang meridians from the hand to the head, those on the three foot yang meridians from the head to the foot, and those on the three foot yin meridians from the foot to the abdomen or chest. Additionally, the acupoints on the conception vessel and the governor vessel are listed from lower to upper. This method of arrangement was previously referred to as "point arrangement along the meridian". However, since the arrangement of the points on the governor vessel does not follow the same direction as the flow of qi and blood, the term "along the meridian" might lead to misunderstandings. Consequently, in this context, the method will be referred to as "point arrangement by meridian". The term "point arrangement along the meridian" will specifically denote the style that is completely consistent with the direction of qi and blood flow.

2. The development of meridian point arrangement

2.1 *The Inner Classic*

Nine Needles and Twelve Yuan-Source Points of *The Spiritual Pivot*: ... There are 27 pathways of qi flowing upward and downward throughout the body. The point where qi begins to emerge is called the Jing-well; where it flows is called the Xing-spring; where it infuses is the Shu-stream; where it moves is termed the Jing-river; and where it enters is known as the He-sea. All 27 pathways of qi pass through the five transport points.

Discussion on Points of *The Spiritual Pivot*: The qi of the lung meridian emerges from Shaoshang (LU11), located on the inner side of the thumb, which is the Jing-well point corresponding to wood. It then flows to Yuji (LU10), situated on the thenar and serving as the Xing-spring point. The qi infuses into Taiyuan (LU9), found in the depression one *cun* posterior to the thenar and identified as the Shu-stream point. It then runs to Jingqu (LU8), located in the middle of the Cunkou where the pulse is always felt and it's the Jing-river point. It enters Chize (LU5), situated at the elbow where the pulse can be palpated and this is the He-sea point. These are the five transport points of the hand Taiyin meridian.

Discussion on the Cave of Qi of *Basic Questions*: There are five lines on the head, with each containing five points, totaling 25 points. Additionally, there are five points located on each side of the spine column, making a total of 10 points...

Discussion on the Mansion of Qi of *Basic Questions*: There're 78 points on the foot Taiyang meridian. Each point is located at the medial end of the two eyebrows...From Weizhong (BL40) downward to the lateral side of the little toe, there are 6 acupoints along this pathway.

As a book with the characteristics of an essay collection, the point arrangements in different sections of *The Inner Classic* vary. Generally, there are two types of arrangements: by region and by meridian, as illustrated in *Discussion on the Cave of Qi* and *Discussion on the Mansion of Qi*, respectively.

In *Discussion on the Mansion of Qi* of *Basic Questions*, the points arranged by meridian primarily include the six yang meridians, the conception vessel, the governor vessel, and the thoroughfare vessel. When listed by meridian, the points of each meridian are then described broadly according to their locations. In *Discussion on Points* of *The Spiritual Pivot*, 11 meridians (excluding the heart meridian) are listed in the order of the zang organs first and then the fu organs. In each meridian, the five transport points are listed in a unidirectional and centripetal sequence. Specifically, regardless of whether the meridian is yin or yang, the five transport points are arranged in the order of Jing-well, Xing-spring, Shu-stream, Jing-river, and He-sea, from the ends of the extremities to the elbow or knee joint.

This arrangement of the five transport points emphasizes the significance of the points located on the distal part of the four limbs, particularly those below the elbows and knees.

KNOWLEDGE DATABASE: CULTURE

The determination of the pronunciation of 荥 (in Xing-spring points)

The corresponding Chinese character for Xing-spring is 荥. In Chinese, it can be pronounced as either xíng or yíng. When pronounced xíng, the character can refer to different meanings. It can refer to an area, such as Xingyang (荥阳), which is named after a marsh called Xing (荥泽). Additionally, it can denote very small water, though this usage is rarely seen in modern Chinese.

When pronounced yíng, the character is even less commonly seen in modern Chinese. However, it can still be found in the name of a place, 荥经 (Yingjing). In classical Chinese, it's used to describe the rise of waves.

The naming of the five transport points is based on analogy. Qi and blood emerge (Jing-well) from the tips, then flow (Xing-spring) and infuse (Shu-stream) through the metacarphalangeal or metatarsophalangeal joints, run (Jing-river) through the wrists or ankles, and then enter (He-sea) the elbows or knees. Qi and blood flow like water, from the small to the large. In the translation, the water metaphor is used. Each type of point is translated using a combination of pinyin and its literal meaning, such as Jing-well points, where "Jing" is the pinyin for 井, meaning well, a shaft sunk into the ground to obtain water. Since 荥 is a polyphonic character, the pronunciation should align with its meaning. The qi and blood here are not abundant, similar to water emerging from a well and forming a spring without any waves. Therefore, it should be read as "Xing", leading to the translation of "Xing-spring points". However, due to certain factors, the translation "Ying-spring points" is often encountered.

2.2 *The Systematic Classic of Acupuncture and Moxibustion*

> *Volume 3*: Part 1: 7 points in total, from the hairline directly above the middle of the nose to the lateral Touwei (ST8)... Part 9: 26 points in total, from three *cun* lateral to the second vertebra to the lateral area below the 21st vertebra on the back... Part 15: 12 points in total from Shufu (KI27), which is 2 *cun* lateral to the conception vessel, downwards to Bulang (KI22)... Part 24: 18 points in total on the hand Taiyin and the arm... including Shaoshang (LU11)... Yuji (LU10)... Taiyuan (LU9)...Jingqu (LU8)... Lieque (LU7)... Kongzui (LU6)... Chize (LU5)... Xiabai (LU4)... and Tianfu (LU3)... Part 25: a total of 16 points on the hand Jueyin pericardium and the arm... Part 26: a total of 16 points on the hand Shaoyin and the arm... Part 27: a total of 28 points on the hand Yangming and the arm...

The Systematic Classic provides a summary of acupoint theory with a clearer and more organized point arrangement compared with *The Inner Classic*. In this book, the points are arranged according to the general line of different body parts: from the head→back→face→neck→shoulder→chest→axilla and lateral thorax→abdomen→upper limbs→lower limbs. On the head, face, and trunk, the points are arranged from top to bottom, and from medial to lateral. In contrast, on the four limbs, the points are organized according to their respective meridians.

In *The Systematic Classic*, the 12 meridians on the four limbs are arranged as follows: three hand ying meridians, three hand yang meridians, three foot yin meridians, and three foot yang meridians. Both the three yin and yang meridians are arranged from medial to lateral. In each meridian, the five transport points located below the elbows or knees, as well as those on the upper arms and thighs, all follow a unidirectional and centripetal pattern. This arrangement of the five transport points is described in *The Inner Classic*.

2.3 The Classified Bright Hall Theory of Huangdi's Inner Classic

> *Preface* : Each of the twelve regular meridians is covered in one volume, and all eight extraordinary vessels are covered in one volume, making a total of 13 volumes.
>
> *Volume 1*: Lung organ... Zhongfu(LU1), Tianfu (LU3), Xiabai (LU4), Chize (LU5), Kongzui (LU6), Lieque (LU7), Jingqu (LU8), Taiyuan (LU9), Yuji (LU10), Shaoshang (LU11).

In Yang Shangshan's *The Classified Bright Hall Theory of Huangdi's Inner Classic*, only the first volume has been preserved. This volume includes the self-preface and the points of the hand Taiyin meridian. The pattern of point arrangement for the other meridians can be inferred from the contents of the hand Taiyin: the points are organized according to the ebb-flow of qi and blood within the meridians, or, in other words, point arrangement along the meridian.

Because the qi and blood in the lung meridian of the hand Taiyin flows from the chest to the hand, in this book, the five transport points are listed not in a centripetal manner but from the proximal to the distal part, as aligning naturally with the flow of qi and blood in the lung meridian. From this, it can be inferred that the arrangement of the other five transport points in the hand-foot and yin-yang meridians in *The Classified Bright Hall Theory of Huangdi's Inner Classic* may vary. Generally, the pattern is centripetal for the hand-yang and foot-yin meridians, and centrifugal for the hand-yin and foot-yang meridians. This arrangement is also known as the circulatory pattern.

2.4 Supplement to "Important Formulas worth a Thousand Gold Pieces"

> *Volume 26*: *No. 1, Methods of Point Locating* (*Juàn Èr Shí Liù · Qǔ Kǒng Xué Fǎ Dì Yī*, 卷二十六·取孔穴法第一): Part 1: 26 points on the face (front side)... Part 5: 6 points located posterior to the ear (back side)... Part 9: 20 points on the ear and neck (lateral side)... Part 11: 7 points directly below the central chest (first line)... Part 19: 10 points on the lung meridian

of the hand Taiyin... Part 20: 20 points on the large intestine meridian of the hand Yangming... Part 21: 8 points on the heart meridian of the hand Shaoyin... Part 22: 9 points on the small intestine meridian of the hand Taiyang... Part 23: 8 points on the pericardium meridian of the hand Jueyin... Part 24: 17 points on the triple energizer meridian of the hand Shaoyang... Part 25: 12 points on the spleen meridian of the foot Taiyin... Part 26: 15 points on the stomach meridian of the foot Yangming... Part 27: 11 points on the liver meridian of the foot Jueyin... Part 28: 15 points on the gallbladder meridian of the foot Shaoyang... Part 29: 11 points on the kidney meridian of the foot Shaoyin... Part 30: 17 points on the bladder meridian of the foot Taiyang...

Supplement to "Important Formulas Worth a Thousand Gold Pieces" is similar to *The Systematic Classic* in that it organizes points on the head and trunk by region, and points on the four limbs by meridian. However, in *Supplement to "Important Formulas Worth a Thousand Gold Pieces"*, the 12 meridians of the four limbs are arranged according to the interior-exterior relationship of the 12 meridians, starting with the hand meridians followed by the foot meridians. Within each meridian, the points are arranged from the tips of the limbs toward the center.

In *Classic of Nourishing Life with Acupuncture and Moxibustion* written during the Southern Song Dynasty, the point arrangement is similar to that found in this book.

2.5 *Arcane Essentials from the Imperial Library*

Volume 39: Preface to the Bright Hall (*Juàn Sān Shí Jiǔ · Míng Táng Xù*, 卷三十九·明堂序): The 12 regular meridians are depicted in five colors, while the 8 extraordinary vessels are shown in green. Although other authors typically illustrate the meridian system using three figures, I will now create 12 figures for each of the 12 regular meridians.

Volume 39: The Bright Hall Theory of Five Zang and Six Fu Organs in Twelve Figures (*Juàn Sān Shí Jiǔ · Shí Èr Shēn Liú Zhù Wǔ Zàng Liù Fǔ Míng Táng*, 卷三十九·十二身流注五脏六腑明堂): The lung meridian figure... The large intestine meridian figure... The liver meridian figure... The gallbladder meridian figure... The spleen meridian figure... The stomach meridian figure... The heart meridian figure... The small intestine meridian figure... The pericardium meridian figure... The kidney meridian figure... The bladder meridian figure... The triple energizer meridian figure...

Arcane Essentials from the Imperial Library organizes the points according to their respective meridians, listing them by meridian. Among the 12 meridians, those with exterior-interior relationships are placed adjacent to each other, though the order of hand and foot meridians may vary. Within each meridian, the points are arranged in a centripetal order, progressing from the tips of the limbs toward the center.

In *Arcane Essentials from the Imperial Library*, the points of the conception vessel are attached to the kidney meridian of foot Shaoyin. The points from Jiuwei (CV15) to Huiyin (CV1) are listed first, starting from top to bottom; then the points from Lianquan (RN23) to Zhongting (RN16), are also arranged from top to bottom. The points of the governor vessel are attached to the bladder meridian of foot Taiyang, extending from Suliao (GV25) on the face down to Changqiang (GV1) on the coccyx.

2.6 *Illustrated Classic of Acupoints on the Bronze Figure*

Volume 1: 22 points in total on both sides of the lung meridian of hand Taiyin... 38 points in total on both sides of the small intestine meridian of hand Taiyang... 40 points in total on both sides of the large intestine meridian of hand Yangming... 26 points in total on both sides of the liver meridian of foot Jueyin... 86 points in total on both sides of the gallbladder meridian of foot Shaoyang...54 points in total on both sides of the kidney meridian of foot Shaoyin...

Volume 2: 18 points in total on both sides of the heart meridian of hand Shaoyin... 18 points in total on both sides of the pericardium meridian of hand Jueyin... 126 points in total on both sides of the bladder meridian of foot Taiyang... 90 points in total on both sides of the stomach meridian of foot Yangming...46 points in total on both sides of the triple energizer meridian of hand Shaoyang... 42 points in total on both sides of the spleen meridian of foot Taiyin... The governor vessel: (points are arranged from the nasal bridge downward, from the forehead upward, from the vertex to the nape of the neck, and downward along the spine)...The conception vessel: (points are arranged in the order of anterior to the cheek, from the jaw downward, along the chest and along the abdominal midline)...

Volume 3: 11 points in total on the midline of the head (both front and back sides)... 16 points in total on both lateral sides of the face...

Volume 4: A total of 111 points on the left, right, and middle regions of the shoulder, upper arm and back... A total of 69 points in the regions of the lateral neck and chest... A total of 87 points in the regions of the abdomen and flank...

Volume 5: 18 points in total on both sides of the lung meridian of hand Taiyin... 18 points in total on both sides of the large intestine meridian of hand Yangming... 18 points in total on both sides of the heart meridian of hand Shaoyin... 16 points in total on both sides of the small intestine of hand Taiyang... 16 points in total on both sides of the pericardium meridian of hand Jueyin... 24 points in total on both sides of the triple energizer meridian of hand Shaoyang...

> 22 points in total on both sides of the liver meridian of foot Jueyin... 28 points in total on both sides of the gallbladder meridian of foot Shaoyang... 22 points in total on both sides of the spleen meridian of foot Taiyin... 30 points in total on both sides of the stomach meridian of foot Yangming... 20 points in total on both sides of the kidney meridian of foot Shaoyin... 36 points in total on both sides of the bladder meridian of foot Taiyang...

The *Illustrated Classic of Acupoints on the Bronze Figure* employs two ways for arranging points: by region and by meridian. In volumes 1 and 2, the points of 14 meridians are organized according to their respective meridians. However, the order of these meridians appears somewhat disorganized, as it doesn't follow the flow of the ying qi. The points of each of the 12 meridians are arranged from the tips of the four limbs towards the head, face or trunk. In contrast, the points for the conception vessel and governor vessel are arranged from the top down.

In volumes 3 to 5, points on the head, face, and trunk are depicted in three figures: the front, back, and lateral sides. They are organized in separate lines according to their regions, listed from top to bottom and from medial to lateral. The 12 regular meridians on the four limbs are listed according to their exterior-interior relationship, with hand meridians preceding foot meridians. Points on each meridian are arranged centripetally, starting from the tips of the four limbs.

2.7 *Comprehensive Recording of Divine Assistance* (*Shèng Jì Zǒng Lù*, 圣济总录)

> *Volume 191:* The lung meridian of hand Taiyin... The large intestine meridian of hand Yangming... The stomach meridian of foot Yangming... The spleen meridian of foot Taiyin... The heart meridian of hand Shaoyin... The small intestine meridian of hand Taiyang... The bladder meridian of foot Taiyang... The kidney meridian of foot Shaoyin... The pericardium meridian of hand Jueyin... The triple energizer meridian of hand Shaoyang... The gallbladder meridian of foot Shaoyang... The liver meridian of foot Jueyin...
>
> *Volume 192:* The governor vessel runs from the head along the spine to enter the sacrum. Its length is 4 *chi* 5 *cun*, and it has a total of 27 points, including Suliao (GV25)... Shuigou (GV26)... Duiduan (GV27)... Yinjiao (GV28)... Shenting (GV24)... Changqiang (GV1)... The conception vessel originates from the uterus and runs upwards to enter the eyes. Its length is 4 *chi* 5 *cun*, and it has a total of 24 points... including Huiyin (CV1)... and Chengjiang (CV24)...

In *Comprehensive Recording of Divine Assistance*, the points of the 14 meridians are arranged according to the 14-meridian circulation. The points of the governor vessel are listed from top to bottom, starting from Shenting (GV24) to Changqiang (GV1), following the four points from Suliao (GV25) to Yinjiao (GV28). Conversely, the points of the conception vessel are listed from bottom to top, beginning at Huiyin (CV1) to Chengjiang (CV24).

KNOWLEDGE DATABASE: LITERATURE

***Comprehensive Recording of Divine Assistance* (*Shèng Jì Zǒng Lù*, 圣济总录)**

Comprehensive Recording of Divine Assistance, a 200-volume medical book, was compiled under the government organization during the Song Dynasty between 1111 and 1117. It was republished twice in later dynasties. The content is derived from medical texts of previous dynasties, folk collections and contributions from doctors. It covers the clinical manifestations and treatments of various diseases.

2.8 *Elucidation on Fourteen Channels*

The Middle Volume: The lung meridian of hand Taiyin has 11 points, including Zhongfu (LU1), Yunmen (LU2), and Tianfu (LU3)... The hand Yangming meridian starts from Shangyang (LI 1)... The foot Yangming meridian has 45 points, including Chengqi (ST1), Sibai (ST2) and Juliao (ST3)... The spleen meridian of foot Taiyin has 21 points, including yinbai (SP1), Dadu (SP2) and Taibai (SP3)... The hand Shaoyin has 9 points, including Jiquan (HT1), Qingling (HT2) and Shaohai (HT3)...The hand Taiyang meridian has 19 points, including Shaoze (SI1), Qiangu (SI2) and Houxi (SI3)...The foot Taiyang meridian has 63 points, including Jingming (BL1), Cuanzhu (BL2) and Qucha (BL4)...The foot Shaoyin meridian has 27 points, including Yongquan (KI1), Rangu (KI2) and Taixi (KI3)...The pericardium meridian of hand Jueyin has 9 points, including Tianchi (PC1), Tianquan (PC2) and Quze (PC3)... The hand Shaoyang meridian has 23 points, including Guanchong (SJ1), Yemen (SJ2) and Zhongzhu (SJ3)... The foot Shaoyang meridian starts with Tongziliao (GB1)... The foot Jueyin meridian has 13 points and starts from Dadun (LR1)... The governor vessel, running along the posterior midline, has 27 points, which start from Changqiang (GV1)... The conception vessel has 24 points, starting from Huiyin (CV1) and running to Qugu (CV2)...

Elucidation on Fourteen Channels follows a pattern of point arrangement by meridian. Unlike the *Comprehensive Recording of Divine Assistance*, where the points of the governor vessel are listed from top to bottom, this book lists them from the bottom up. This pattern of point arrangement is commonly used in modern times. According to the notes at the end of the middle volume of *Elucidation on Fourteen Channels*, this arrangement actually originated from *Illustrated Point Location along Meridians from the Gold-Orchid Chamber*, which was written and edited in 1303 by Hu Gong Tai, an acupuncture professor form the Yuan Dynasty. Gao Wu noted that the author's name was "Hu Tai Bi Lie".

In the Ming Dynasty, *A Collection of Gems in Acupuncture and Moxibustion* (*Zhēn Jiǔ Jù Yīng*, 针灸聚英) also adopted this pattern of arrangement.

Thereafter, the point arrangement pattern in *Pictorial Appendices to "The Classified Classic"* (*Lèi Jīng Tú Yì*, 类经图翼) from the Ming Dynasty and *Essential Teachings on Acupuncture and Moxbustion* of *Golden Mirror of the Medical Tradition* (*Yī Zōng Jīn Jiàn · Cì Jiǔ Xīn Fǎ Yào Jué*, 医宗金鉴·刺灸心法要诀) from the Qing Dynasty is largely consistent with that of *Elucidation on Fourteen Channels*, except for the reversed order of the governor vessel and conception vessel.

KNOWLEDGE DATABASE: LITERATURE

A Collection of Gems in Acupuncture and Moxibustion (*Zhēn Jiǔ Jù Yīng*, 针灸聚英)

A Collection of Gems in Acupuncture and Moxibustion, written by Gao Wu, is a 4-volume work on acupuncture and moxibustion published in 1529 during the Ming Dynasty. The book introduces basic theories of meridians and acupoints, while the subsequent volumes compile various theories, techniques, and treatment methods developed in medical texts following *The Inner Classic* and *The Classic of Questioning*.

Gao Wu respected *The Inner Classic* and *The Classic of Questioning*, believing that their theories would endure through generations without any disadvantage. In this book, he evaluated the collected contents based on the principles established in these foundational texts.

Pictorial Appendices to "The Classified Classic" (*Lèi Jīng* Tú Yì, 类经图翼)

Pictorial Appendices to "The Classified Classic" is an 11-volume sequel written by Zhang Jiebin to complement his earlier work, *The Classified Classic*, during the Ming Dynasty. The book uses diagrams to address the shortcomings in the annotations in *The Classified Classic*, hence the name "Pictorial Appendices".

KNOWLEDGE DATABASE: HISTORY

The Qing Dynasty

The Qing Dynasty (清朝、清代) was the last imperial dynasty of China, ruling from 1644 to 1911. It succeeded the Ming Dynasty and was followed by the Republic of China period. The Qing Dynasty was led by the Manchus, a minority ethnic group.

KNOWLEDGE DATABASE: LITERATURE

***Essential Teachings on Acupuncture and Moxibustion* of *Golden Mirror of the Medical Tradition* (*Yī Zōng Jīn Jiàn · Cì Jiǔ Xīn Fǎ Yào Jué*, 医宗金鉴 · 刺灸心法要诀)**

Golden Mirror of the Medical Tradition is a comprehensive medical series published in 1742 during the Qing Dynasty, with Wu Qian and others serving as the chief editors. Organized by the government, the series consists of 90 volumes, which are divided into 15 fascicules. The fascicule on acupuncture and moxibustion is called *Essential Teachings on Acupuncture and Moxibustion*. Comprising 8 volumes (volumes 79–86), it summarizes and discusses the basic theories and clinical diagnosis of acupuncture and moxibustion, through seven-character song verses.

3. The order of the arrangement of meridians and points and other acumox theories

3.1 The arrangement of the five transport points and the theories of branch-root and original-terminal

Origin and Terminal of *The Spiritual Pivot* (*Líng Shū · Gēn Jié*, 灵枢 · 根结): The origin of Taiyang is at Zhiyin (BL67), and its terminal is at the life gate (命门 in character, referring to eyes)... The origin of Yangming is at Lidui (ST45), and its terminal is in the throat... The origin of Shaoyang is at Qiaoyin (GB44), and its terminal is in the ear... The origin of Taiyin is at Yinbai (SP1), and its terminal is in the stomach. The origin of Shaoyin is at Yongquan (KI1), and its terminal is beneath the tongue. The origin of Jueyin is at Dadun (LR1), and its terminal is in the private parts.

Origin and Terminal of *The Spiritual Pivot*: The foot Taiyang originates from Zhiyin (BL67), flows to Jinggu (BL64), infuses into Kunlun (BL60), and then enters to Tianzhu (BL10) and Feiyang (BL58). The foot Shaoyang originates from Qiaoyin (GB44), flows to Qiuxu (GB40), infuses into Yangfu (GB38), and enters Tianrong (SI17) and Guangming (GB37). The foot Yangming originates from Lidui (ST45), flows to Chongyang (ST42), infuses into Xialing (ST36), and enters Renyin (ST9) and Fenglong (ST40). The hand Taiyang originates from Shaoze (SI1), flows to Yanggu (SI5), infuses into Xiaohai (SI8), and enters Tianchuang (SI16) and Zhizheng (SI7). The hand Shaoyang originates from Guanchong (SJ1), flows to Yangchi (SJ4), infuses into Zhigou (SJ6), and enters Tianyou (SJ16) and Waiguan (SJ5). The hand

Yangming originates from Shangyang (LI1), flows to Hegu (LI4), infuses into Yangxi (LI5), and enters Futu (LI18) and Pianli (LI6).

Wei Qi of *The Spiritual Pivot*: The root of the foot Taiyang is located 5 *cun* superior to the heel, while its branch is located in the eye... The root of the foot Shaoyang is found at Qiaoyin (GB44), with its branch located in the area anterior to the ear... The root of the foot Shaoyin is positioned 3 *cun* inferior to the medial malleolus, and its branch is located at the back-Shu point and two vessels beneath the tongue. The root of the foot Jueyin is located around 5 *cun* superior to Xingjian (LR2), with its branch located at the back-Shu point. The root of the foot Yangming is at Lidui (ST45), and its branch is found in Renying (ST9), the cheek and the place lateral to the throat. The root of the foot Taiyin is 4 *cun* anterior and superior to Zhongfeng (LR4), with its branch located at the back-Shu point and the root of the tongue. The root of the hand Taiyang is located at the area posterior to the lateral malleolus, with its branch located 1 *cun* superior to the eye. The root of the hand Shaoyang is found 2 *cun* superior to the region between the litter finger and the ring finger, while its branch is located at the posterosuperior corner of the ear and the region inferior to the outer canthus. The root of the hand Yangming is located in the area extending from the elbow up to Bie Yang, and its branch is situated on the forehead, above Qian Shang. The root of the hand Taiyin is found at Cunkou, and the branch is located in the arteries in the armpit. The root of the hand Shaoyin is located at the tip of the pisiform bone of the hand, with its branch found at the back-Shu point. The root of the hand pericardium is situated 2 *cun* posterior to the wrist between the two tendons, while its branch is located at 3 *cun* inferior to the armpit.

In early literature, the arrangement of the five transport points was consistently toward the center. However, after the *Comprehensive Recording of Divine Assistance* from the Song Dynasty, the arrangement of the five transport points was organized according to the ebb-flow of qi and blood through the 12 meridians. This arrangement follows two directions: either toward the center or away from the center.

The order of the five transport points—Jing-well, Xing-spring, Shu-stream, Jing-river, and He-sea—demonstrates the characteristic that the qi and blood of each meridian increase in volume as they flow from the tip of the limb toward the center. This arrangement aligns with the origin-terminal theory, where the origins of the six foot meridians are in the four limbs, and the terminals are in the head, chest, and abdomen. It also corresponds with the originate-flow-infuse-enter theory, which states that the six yang meridians originate from the Jing-well points on the four limbs and ascend to the neck points. It also adheres to the root-branch theory from *The Inner Classic*, which states that the 12 meridians have their roots in the lower parts of the four limbs and their branches extend to the head, face, chest, and back. This illustrates the distant effect of the points on the four limbs on the head and trunk, and the foundational relationship between them.

KNOWLEDGE DATABASE

Origin and Terminal of *The Spiritual Pivot* (*Líng Shū · Gēn Jié*, 灵枢 · 根结): The 5th chapter of the *Ling Shu*. It primarily discusses the origins and terminals of the meridians.

3.2 The point arrangement of the conception vessel and the governor vessel

The conception vessel and the governor vessel are located on the head, face, and trunk. In *The Systematic Classic of Acupuncture and Moxibustion, Supplement to "Important Formulas Worth a Thousand Gold Pieces"*, and *Classic of Nourishing Life with Acupuncture and Moxibustion*, the points on the head, face, and trunk are arranged by region from top to bottom. Accordingly, the points of the conception and governor vessels are also listed from top to bottom.

In the books that adopt point arrangement by meridian, the points of the governor vessel appear before those of the conception vessel prior to *A Collection of Gems in Acupuncture and Moxibustion*. However, in subsequent works such as *Pictorial Appendices to "The Classified Classic"* and *Essential Teachings on Acupuncture and Moxibustion* of *Golden Mirror of the Medical Tradition*, the order of the two vessels is reversed.

Regarding the points of the governor vessel, in books that adopt a meridian-based point arrangement, they're listed from the head and face down to the coccyx in the *Illustrated Classic of Acupoints on the Bronze Figure* and *Comprehensive Recording of Divine Assistance*. However, in *Elucidation on Fourteen Channels*, the points are listed from the bottom up. Regarding the points of the conception vessel, in books that use a meridian-based point arrangement, they're listed from the top down in the *Illustrated Classic of Acupoints on the Bronze Figure*. However, following the *Comprehensive Recording of Divine Assistance*, the points began to be listed from the bottom up.

According to the ebb-flow order of ying qi, the governor vessel runs downward while the conception vessel runs upward. The point arrangement by meridian pattern in the *Comprehensive Recording of Divine Assistance* aligns with this principle of yin ascending and yang descending.

4. Note

In historical medical literature, there is inconsistency in the point arrangement for the large intestine meridian of hand Yangming, the stomach meridian of foot Yangming, the spleen meridian of foot

Taiyin, the small intestine meridian of hand Taiyang, the bladder meridian of foot Taiyang, the kidney meridian of foot Shaoyin, the triple energizer meridian of hand Shaoyang, and the gallbladder meridian of foot Shaoyang. This situation is caused by various factors, such as errors in copying, differences in meridian attribution, and varying understandings. It's difficult to draw a definitive conclusion until the meridians and their points can be understood objectively.

The patterns of the meridian point arrangement reflect different acupuncture theories. The arrangement of points on the fourteen meridians has been repeatedly summarized in ancient medical texts, leading to the development of the modern pattern of point arrangement for the fourteen meridians. In other words, with the exception of the acupoints on the governor vessel, which are not arranged according to the direction of qi and blood flow, the order of the other meridians and the arrangement of their points are generally consistent with the direction of qi and blood flow. The theories of branch-root, origin-terminal, and originate-flow-infuse-enter from *The Inner Classic* are only reflected in the unidirectional and centripetal arrangement of the five transport points: Jing-well, Xing-spring, Shu-stream, Jing-river, and He-sea points.

Reflections

What is the guiding significance of the point arrangement by meridian and the point arrangement by region for clinical practice?

Terms and Synonyms

(1) History, culture and people

Term	Chinese	Explanations
The Qing Dynasty	清朝、清代	The last imperial dynasty from 1644–1911
Polyphonic character	多音字	Chinese characters with more than two pronunciations
Gao Wu	高 武	The author of *A Collection of Gems in Acupuncture and Moxibustion*
Wu Qian	吴 谦	The author of *Golden Mirror of the Medical Tradition*

(2) Meridians and points

Term	Synonym	Chinese
Root-flow-infuse-enter theory	Gen-Liu-Zhu-Ru theory	根溜注入
Point arrangement along the meridian		循经列穴

(continued)

Term	Synonym	Chinese
Jing-well points	Well point	井 穴
Xing-spring points	Ying-spring points, Brook point	荥 穴
Shu-stream points	Stream point	输 穴
Jing-river points	River point	经 穴
He-sea points	Sea point	合 穴
Back-Shu points	Transport point	背俞穴

(3) Book names

Term	Synonym	Chinese
Comprehensive Recording of Divine Assistance	*Sheng Ji Zong Lu*	圣济总录
A Collection of Gems in Acupuncture and Moxibustion	*Zhen Jiu Ju Ying*	针灸聚英
Pictorial Appendices to "The Classified Classic"	*Lei Jing Tu Yi*	类经图翼
Golden Mirror of the Medical Tradition	*Yi Zong Jin Jian*	医宗金鉴

(4) Chapters of *The Inner Classic*

The Spiritual Pivot

Term	Synonym	Chinese
Origin and Terminal	*Gen Jie*	根 结

Topic 5

The Yuan-Source Points

1. The general knowledge of Yuan-source point

Each of the 12 regular meridians has a point located near the wrist or ankle joints. This position is where the original qi of the zang-fu organs resides and is known as a Yuan-source point. Collectively, these Yuan-source points are referred to as the "Twelve Yuan" (Table 1–3). "Yuan" denotes origin and primary qi, which is the fundamental energy of human life.

Table 1–3　The Yuan-source points of the twelve meridians

Three Yin of Hand		**Three Yang of Hand**		**Three Yang of Foot**		**Three Yin of Foot**	
Lung	LU9	Large intestine	LI4	Stomach	ST42	Spleen	SP3
Heart	HT7	Small intestine	SI4	Bladder	BL64	Kidney	KI3
Pericardium	PC7	Sanjiao	TE4	Gallbladder	GB40	Liver	LR3

According to Table 1–3, the Yuan-source points of the yin meridians correspond to the Shu-stream points among the five transport points. This is illustrated by the statement that "yin meridians use Shu-stream points as Yuan-source points". In contrast, yang meridians have a distinct Yuan-source point in addition to the five transport points.

The Yuan-source points can be used to diagnose and treat diseases of the five zang and six fu organs.

2. The development of the Yuan-source points

2.1 *Nine Needles and Twelve Yuan-Source Points* of *The Spiritual Pivot*

The five zang organs have the six fu organs exteriorly, and the six fu organs have twelve Yuan-source points exteriorly. The twelve Yuan-source points come out at the four joints, and the four joints control the cure of the five zang organs. When the five zang organs are affected by disease, the twelve Yuan-source points should be used for treatment. Through the twelve Yuan-source points, the five zang organs impart qi and flavour to the three hundred and sixty-five sections of the body. When the five zang organs are diseased, the reactions will manifest at these twelve Yuan-source points. Each of the twelve Yuan-source points has its own specific source. Therefore, when the Yuan-source points are thoroughly understood, and reactions are observed, the problems of the five zang organs can be identified.

Shaoyin in yang corresponds to the lung, with its Yuan-source point located at Taiyuan (LU9), which is bilateral. Taiyang in yang corresponds to the heart, with its Yuan-source point located at Daling (PC7), which is also bilateral. Shaoyang in yin corresponds to the liver, with its Yuan-source point located at Taichong (LR3), which is bilateral. Zhiyin in yin corresponds to the spleen, with its Yuan-source point located at Taibai (SP3), also bilateral. Taiyin in yin corresponds to the kidney, with its Yuan-source point located at Taixi (KI3), which is bilateral. The Yuan-source point for Gao is located at Jiuwei (CV15), which is a singular point. The Yuan-source point for Huang is found at Boyang (CV6), which is also singular. All twelve Yuan-source points play a crucial role in treating the five zang organs and six fu organs when they are diseased.

Nine Needles and Twelve Yuan-Source Points is the first chapter of *The Spiritual Pivot*. The excerpt above describes the twelve Yuan-source points located around the elbows, knees, chest, and navel, and explains the pathological connections between the twelve Yuan-source points and zang-fu organs.

The twelve Yuan-source points can be referred to as the "Yuan-source points of the five zang organs". According to the definition, they are primarily related to the five zang organs and the chest-abdomen. As stated, "Through the twelve Yuan-source points, the five zang organs impart qi and flavour to the three hundred and sixty-five sections of the body". Its locations are described as "come out at the four joints"; and it consists of twelve points. However, while the number of points is the same as in modern terminology, their specific contents do not fully align with those of the contemporary system. (Table 1–4)

Table 1–4 The Yuan-source points of the five zang organs

Five Zang Organs & Gao, Huang	Yuan-Source Point	Number of Point
Lung	Taiyuan (LU9)	2
Heart	Daling (PC7)	2
Liver	Taichong (LR3)	2
Spleen	Taibai (SP3)	2
Kidney	Taixi (KI3)	2
Gao (diaphragm)	Jiuwei (CV15)	1
Huang (omentum)	Boyang (CV6)	1

It should to be noted that Daling (PC7) belongs to the pericardium meridian. The reason it is listed as the Yuan-source point for the heart here is that in *The Inner Classic*, the heart is considered the sovereign organ, which can't be attacked by pathogenic factors, as it would lead to death. Thus, "all the evils affecting the heart are actually present in the pericardium." This means that the pericardium bears the evils for the heart, and its points can be used to treat heart conditions. This explains why the five transport points and Yuan-source points of the heart mentioned in *The Inner Classic* are actually the points of the pericardium meridian of the hand Jueyin.

The Yuan-source points of the five zang organs can be used for both diagnosis and treatment. As stated in the article, "When the five zang organs are diseased, the reactions will be manifested at the twelve Yuan-source points. Each of the twelve Yuan-source points has its own specific source. Therefore, when the Yuan-source points are thoroughly understood, and reactions are observed, the problems of the five zang organs can be identified." For treatment, it's suggested, "When the five zang organs are diseased, the twelve Yuan-source points should be used for treatment."

KNOWLEDGE DATABASE: CULTURE

Gao, Huang, Gaohuang & Two Kids (膏 | 肓 | 膏肓 | 二竖)

Gao, originally meaning oil or fat, refers to the fat around the heart. However, in the term Gaohuang (膏肓), the character 膏 is a typo. The correct character should be Ge (鬲), which is equivalent to Ge (膈) in modern usage, meaning diaphragm.

Huang (肓) refers to the omentum, a fold of peritoneum that supports the viscera.

Gaohuang (膏肓) has two meanings in TCM. Its literal meaning is the area between the heart and the diaphragm, which is considered the deepest area of the body and beyond the reach of most treatments.

Additionally, Gaohuang refers to an acupoint on the bladder meridian of the foot Taiyang, known as BL43.

For the first meaning of Gaohuang, there's a Chinese idiom used to describe a very serious disease: "病入膏肓", meaning the disease has reached the area of Gaohuang. The idiom originates from a story set in the Spring and Autumn Period, in which a king had a disease and sent for a doctor, Huan. Before the arrival of the doctor, the king had a dream in which two kids were discussing the coming doctor. One said, "A good doctor will come and do harm to us. How can we run from him?" The other replied, "We can move to the area above Huang, but below Gao. What can he do with us?" Doctor Huan arrived and told the king, "Your disease can't be cured. It's above Huang, but below Gao, and can neither be attacked nor reached. The medicine is useless. I can do nothing."

Two kids ("Er Shu" in pin yin, 二竖) is an allusion derived from the aforementioned story. In China, when someone has a serious illness and wishes to express it indirectly in a classic and literary manner, he might say: "I'm troubled by two kids."

2.2 *Discussion on Points* of *The Spiritual Pivot*

> The bladder meridian... passes through Jinggu (BL64)... which is the Yuan-source point... .
>
> The gallbladder meridian... passes through Qiuxu (GB40)... which is the Yuan-source point... .
>
> The stomach meridian... passes through Chongyang (ST42)... which is the Yuan-source point... .
>
> The Sanjiao meridian... passes through Yangchi (TE4)... which is the Yuan-source point... .
>
> The small intestine meridian... passes through Wangu (SI4)... which is the Yuan-source point....
>
> The large intestine meridian... passes through Hegu (LI4)... which is the Yuan-source point....

Discussion on Points of *The Spiritual Pivot* introduces the five transport points of the five zang and six fu organs. It states that there are "five times five is twenty-five points" for the yin meridians and "six times six is thirty-six points" for the yang meridians. The "five times five is twenty-five points" for yin meridians refers to the Jing-well, Xing-spring, Shu-stream, Jing-river, and He-sea points of the lung, heart, liver, spleen, and kidney. In contrast, the "six times six is thirty-six points" for yang meridians includes the Jing-well, Xing-spring, Shu-stream, Yuan-source, Jing-river, and He-sea points of the bladder, gallbladder, stomach, Sanjiao, small intestine, and large intestine. In other words, *Discussion on Points* of *The Spiritual Pivot* expands the concept of Yuan-source points for the yang meridians.

2.3 *Division of One Day into Four Seasons Conforming to Qi* of *The Spiritual Pivot* (*Líng Shū · Shùn Qì Yī Rì Fēn Wéi Sì Shí*, 灵枢·顺气一日分为四时)

> Huang Di asked, "How are all the Yuan-source points included into the system to ensure that the six types of points correspond to the five seasons?" Qi Bo replied, "The Yuan-source point is the only type that doesn't correspond to the five seasons. It's merged with the Jing-river point, and together they complete the total number; that is, six times six equals thirty-six points."

In *Division of One Day into Four Seasons Conforming to Qi* of *The Spiritual Pivot*, the seasons of spring, summer, long summer, autumn, and winter are aligned with the five transport points: Jing-well, Xing-spring, Shu-stream, Jing-river, and He-sea, respectively. This arrangement is discussed in the topic "five transport points controlled by five changes". For the six fu organs, in addition to the five transport points, there is also the Yuan-source point. Regarding the alignment of the Yuan-source point with the five seasons, the explanation in the *Division of One Day into Four Seasons Conforming to Qi* is that "it's merged with the Jing-river point". This means that the Yuan-source point is categorized together with the Jing-river point, and they share the same characteristics. As a result, the six types of points can correspond with the five seasons.

KNOWLEDGE DATABASE: LITERATURE

Division of One Day into Four Seasons Conforming to Qi of *The Spiritual Pivot* (*Líng Shū · Shùn Qì Yī Rì Fēn Wéi Sì Shí*, 灵枢·顺气一日分为四时): The 44th chapter of the *Ling Shu*. It discusses the patterns and principles of changes in disease conditions over the course of a day, as well as the reasons why diseases do not change in severity according to the aforementioned patterns. It also introduces the significance of the five changes, including the clinical applications.

2.4 *Invasion of Evils* of *The Spiritual Pivot*

> Huang Di asked: "The Shaoyin meridian is the only one without any points; does that mean it's protected from all illnesses?" Qi Bao answered: "The external meridian can be affected and the zang won't be diseased. Therefore, in such a case, the point located at the tip of the pointed bone superior to the palm can be used. "

According to *Invasions of Evils*, while the heart, as a zang organ, is not directly affected by external evils and does not contract diseases, its meridian can still be influenced by such factors. In other words, "the external meridian can be affected, but the zang organ itself won't be diseased." Diseases affecting the external meridian of the heart can be treated with the point at the "tip of the pointed bone superior to the palm", which is the same as Shenmen (HT7).

2.5 *The 62nd Issue* of *The Classic of Questioning* (*Nàn Jīng · Liù Shí Èr Nàn*, 难经 · 六十二难)

> Each zang organ has five points, including the Jing-well point and the Xing-spring point, among others. However, each fu organ has six points. Why is this the case?
>
> Well, fu organs correspond to yang and are associated with Sanjiao, which flows through all yang areas; therefore, an additional point, known as the Yuan-source point, is established. As a result, each fu organ has six points. This is because fu organs share their qi with the Sanjiao.

The chapter *Nine Needles and Twelve Yuan-Source Points* in *The Spiritual Pivot* states that "each of the five zang organs has five points, and five times five is twenty-five points; each of the six fu organs has six points, and six times six is thirty-six points". Regarding this statement, the *Sixty-two Issue* explains that the five zang organs have five transport points: the Jing-well, Xing-spring, Shu-stream, Jing-river, and He-sea points. In contrast, each of the six fu organs has an additional Yuan-source point, in addition to the five transport points.

The reason for the extra Yuan-source point in addition to the five transport points in the yang meridians of the six fu organs is based on the theory that the Sanjiao flows through all yang areas. Since the qi of the six fu organs communicate with that of the Sanjiao, a Yuan-source point is established at the location where the Sanjiao passes through each of the yang meridians of the six fu organs.

KNOWLEDGE DATABASE: LITERATURE

The 62nd Issue of *The Classic of Questioning* (*Nàn Jīng · Liù Shí Èr Nàn,* 难经 · 六十二难): The 62nd issue of *The Classic of Questioning*. It explains why the fu organs have an additional Yuan-source point.

2.6 *The 66th Issue* of *The Classic of Questioning* (*Nàn Jīng · Liù Shí Liù Nàn*, 难经 · 六十六难)

According to the Classic, the Yuan-source point of the lung is located at Taiyuan (LU9); the Yuan-source point of the heart is at Daling (PC7); the Yuan-source point of the liver is at Taichong (LR3); the Yuan-source point of the spleen is at Taibai (SP3); the Yuan-source point of the kidney is at Taixi (KI3); the Yuan-source of Shaoyin is at the pointed bone (HT7); the Yuan-source of gallbladder is at Qiuxu (GB40); the Yuan-source of stomach is at Chongyang (ST42); the Yuan-source of Sanjiao is at Yangchi (TE4); the Yuan-source of bladder is at Jinggu (BL64); the Yuan-source of large intestine is at Hegu (LI4); the Yuan-source of small intestine is at Wangu (SI4). All twelve meridians use the Shu-stream points as their Yuan-source points. What's the reason for this?

Well, the points of the five zang organs are located where the Sanjiao passes and where qi lingers.

Why are the points through which the Sanjiao flows called Yuan-source points?

Well, the dynamic qi located below the navel and between the kidneys is considered the essence of human life and the root of the twelve meridians, which is why it's referred to as the "original" qi. The Sanjiao, as the special envoy of the original qi, governs the circulations of the three types of qi throughout the five zang and the six fu organs. The term "Yuan-source" is an honorific title for the Sanjiao, so the locations where it resides are referred to as Yuan-source points. These points can be used in the treatment of both conditions affecting the five zang organs and the six fu organs.

In the chapter *Nine Needles and Twelve Yuan-Source Points* in *The Spiritual Pivot*, the Yuan-source points for the five zang organs, chest, and abdomen are introduced. In *Discussion on Points* of *The Spiritual Pivot*, the Yuan-source points for the six fu organs are discussed. In *Invasion of Evils* of *The Spiritual Pivot*, the "tip of the pointed bone" which is used to treat diseases of the Shaoyin meridian, is introduced. In *The 66th Issue* of *The Classic of Questioning*, these concepts are combined, leading to the formation of the Yuan-source points for the twelve meridians. Additionally, the theory regarding yin meridians, which states that the Shu-stream point should be used as the Yuan-source point, is also proposed.

In addition, *The 66th Issue* of *The Classic of Questioning*- provides a further explanation of the statement from *The 62nd Issue* of *The Classic of Questioning* which notes that "Sanjiao flows through all yang areas; therefore, an additional point, known as the Yuan-source point, is established". It also integrates the Yuan-source points with the Yuan-source qi (original qi) below the navel and between the kidneys. This issue points out that the Yuan-source qi is the root of life, and it can only be distributed throughout the body with the guidance of the Sanjiao. In other words, the Sanjiao acts as the special envoy of Yuan-source qi. Consequently, the locations where the qi of the Sanjiao lingers is designated as the Yuan-source point.

The 66th Issue of *The Classic of Questioning* also emphasizes the therapeutic significance of the Yuan-source points, noting that diseases of the five zang and six fu organs can be treated using these points.

The Classic of Questioning defines the basic connotation of the Yuan-source point.

KNOWLEDGE DATABASE: LITERATURE

The 66th Issue of *The Classic of Questioning* (*Nàn Jīng · Liù Shí Liù Nàn,* 难经·六十六难): The 66th issue of *The Classic of Questioning*. It introduces the 12 Yuan-source points and explains the rationale behind their naming.

2.7 *The Systematic Classic of Acupuncture and Moxibustion*

Volume 3: Part 25, 16 points in total of the hand Jueyin pericardium and the arm of *The Systematic Classic of Acupuncture and Moxibustion*: (*Zhēn Jiǔ Jiǎ Yǐ Jīng · Juàn Sān · Shǒu Jué Yīn Xīn Zhǔ Jí Bì Fán Yī Shí Liù Xué Dì Èr Shí Wǔ,* 针灸甲乙经·卷三·手厥阴心主及臂凡一十六穴第二十五): ... Daling (PC7) is associated with the earth. It's located in the depression between the two tendons superior to the palm, where the pericardium meridian of the hand infuses. It's classified as the Shu-stream point.

Volume 3: Part 26, 16 points in total of the hand Shaoyin and the arm of *The Systematic Classic of Acupuncture and Moxibustion* (*Zhēn Jiǔ Jiǎ Yǐ Jīng · Juàn Sān · Shǒu Shǎo Yīn Jí Bì Fán Yī Shí Liù Xué Dì Èr Shí Liù,* 针灸甲乙经·卷三·手少阴及臂凡一十六穴第二十六): ... Shenmen (HT7) is associated with the earth. It is also known by its aliases Duichong and Zhongdu. It's located in the depression at the tip of the pointed bone superior to the palm, where the hand Shaoyin meridian infuses. It's classified as the Shu-stream point.

In *The Systematic Classic of Acupuncture and Moxibustion*, the five transport points of the hand Shaoyin meridian are clearly listed, as Shenmen (HT7) identified as its Shu-stream point. According to the principle of using the Shu-stream point as the Yuan-source point, Shenmen serves as the Yuan-source point for the heart.

Since the points of the heart meridian are listed alongside those of other meridians, the points of the pericardium meridian can be categorized under their own meridian. The five transport points and the Yuan-source points of the heart meridian, as described in *The Inner Classic*, are classified under the pericardium meridian in *The Systematic Classic of Acupuncture and Moxibustion*. The modern concept of Yuan-source points is essentially defined by their names, numbers, and connotations.

2.8 *Important Formulas worth a Thousand Gold Pieces*

> *Volume 29: Part 2, The Flow of Three Yin and Three Yang* of *Important Formulas Worth a Thousand Gold Pieces for Emergency* (*Bèi Jí Qiān Jīn Yào Fāng · Juàn Èr Shí Jiǔ · Sān Yīn Sān Yáng Liú Zhù Dì Èr*, 备急千金要方·卷二十九·三阴三阳流注第二): For all points, the following terms are used: the point where qi starts to emerge is called the Jing-well point; the point where qi starts to flow is called the Xing-spring point; the point where qi infuses is called the Shu-stream point; the point where qi passes through is called the Yuan-source point; the point where qi runs is called the Jing-river point; and the point where qi enters is called the He-sea point. ... The qi of the lung meridian emerges at Shaoshang (LU11), the Jing-well point, flows to Yuji (LU10), the Xing-spring point, infuses into Daquan (LU9), the Shu-stream point, passes through Lieque (LU7), the Yuan-source point, runs to Jingqu (LU8), the Jing-river point, and finally enters Chize (LU5), the He-sea point.
>
> *Volume 26: Part 1, Methods of Point Location* of *Supplement to "Important Formulas Worth a Thousand Gold Pieces"* (*Qiān Jīn Yì Fāng · Juàn Èr Shí Liù · Qǔ Kǒng Xué Fǎ Dì Yī*, 千金翼方·卷二十六·取孔穴法第一): The lung meridian of the hand Taiyin falls under the zang organ category. It emerges from Shaoshang (LU11), the Jing-well point, flows to Yuji (LU10), the Xing-spring point, infuses into Daquan (LU9), the Shu-stream point, passes through Lieque (LU7), the Yuan-source point, runs to Jingqu (LU8), the Jing-river point, and finally enters Chize (LU5), the He-sea point.

The Flow of Three Yin and Three Yang in *Important Formulas Worth a Thousand Gold Pieces for Emergency* describes the basic definitions of the five transport points and the Yuan-source points, and lists them individually. In *Methods of Point Location* from *Supplement to "Important Formulas Worth a Thousand Gold Pieces"*, the five transport points, Yuan-source points, and front-Mu and back-Shu points are all listed, with the lung meridian being used as an example to explain the attributes of each point. In *Important Formulas Worth a Thousand Gold Pieces*, the Yuan-source point for the yin meridian is no longer the Shu-stream point. Instead, there is a separate, independent Yuan-source point located elsewhere (Table 1–5).

Table 1–5 The Yuan-source points of the twelve meridians in *Important Formulas Worth a Thousand Gold Pieces*

Three Yin of Hand		Three Yang of Hand		Three Yang of Foot		Three Yin of Foot	
Hand Taiyin meridian	Lieque (LU7)	Hand Yangming meridian	Hegu (LI4)	Foot Yangming meridian	Chongyang (ST42)	Foot Taiyin meridian	Gongsun (SP4)
Peridium collateral meridian	Neiguan (PC6)	Hand Shaoyang meridian	Yangchi (TE4)	Foot Shaoyang meridian	Qiuxu (GB40)	Foot Jueyin meridian	Zhongfeng (LR4)
Hand Shaoyin meridian	Tongli (HT5)	Hand Taiyang meridian	Wangu (SI4)	Foot Taiyang meridian	Jinggu (BL64)	Foot Shaoyin meridian	Shuiquan (KI5)

As shown in Table 1–5, the Yuan-source points of the yang meridians in *Important Formulas Worth a Thousand Gold Pieces* still adhere to the theory presented in *The Inner Classic*. However, for the three yin meridians of the hand and the foot Taiyin meridian, the Luo-connecting point is used as the Yuan-source point. In the foot Jueyin meridian, the Jing-river point Zhongfeng (LR4) from the five transport points is designated as the Yuan-source point, while in the foot Shaoyin meridian, the Xi-cleft point Shuiquan (KI5) serves as the Yuan-source point.

The preface to the *Three-Figure Picture of The Bright Hall* at the beginning of volume 29 of *Important Formulas Worth a Thousand Gold Pieces for Emergency* states that it "uses the newly compiled book by Zhen Quan and others as the standard". The preface to volume 26 of *Supplement to "Important Formulas Worth a Thousand Gold Pieces"* also states that "the points used for acupuncture and moxibustion are all determined according to *The Picture of the Bright Hall* by Mr. Zhen". Therefore, this practice of using the Luo-connecting point, the Jing-river point, and similar points as the Yuan-source point may originate from *The Bright Hall*, compiled by Zhen Quan. However, since it differs from the theories in *The Inner Classic* or *The Classic of Questioning*, its adoption has been limited.

KNOWLEDGE DATABASE: CULTURE

Taiyuan (太渊) and Daquan (大泉): Homophonic substitution (通假), taboo substitution (避讳)

Taiyuan, coded LU9, is the pinyin for 太渊, the ninth point on the lung meridian. In ancient literature, it's also written as 大渊, which is pronounced Dayuan. The characters Tai (太) and Da (大) are interchangeable, meaning they can be read and understood as the same even though they're different characters. In this case,

Tai and Da both mean great or big and can both be read as Tai. This practice is known as homophonic substitution, which refers to the interchangeable and borrowed usage of Chinese characters, using words with similar or identical sounds to substitute the original characters.

After the beginning of the Tang Dynasty (618–907) , 渊 began to be written as 泉. This change is attributed to a cultural practice known as taboo substitution, which refers to the phenomenon where the names of emperors or respected figures should not be used directly either in writing or speech to show respect and authority. In such cases, other words or characters were used as substitutes to replace those in the original names.

KNOWLEDGE DATABASE: PEOPLE

Zhen Quan (甄权)

Zhen Quan (c. 541–c. 643) took up the study of medicine because of his mother's illness and became a renowned physician during the Tang Dynasty, particularly excelling in acupuncture and moxibustion. His works primarily focused on acupuncture, including illustrations of meridians and acupoints in a work known as *The Picture of the Bright Hall.* He was also renowned for his revision of acupuncture theory, which was commissioned by the emperor. Although none of his books have survived, they were referenced by other physicians, such as Sun Simiao, in their own writings.

3. Note

The origins of the Yuan-source points for the yin and yang meridians differ. In the development of these points, there are variations in their origins, implications, and functions. The Yuan-source points of the five zang organs, as described in *Nine Needles and Twelve Yuan-Source Points* are all named using terms like "Great" (太, Tai) or "Big" (大, Da), which reflects the importance that ancients practitioners placed on these acupoints and underscores their crucial role in diagnosis and treatment.

Reflections

Are there any differences in the application of the Yuan-source points of the yin and yang meridians in clinical diagnosis and treatment? Please conduct a preliminary evaluation and analysis based on a literature review of modern clinical research.

Terms and Synonyms

(1) History, culture and people

Term	Chinese	Explanations
Gaohuang	膏 肓	The deepest area in the body
Er Shu Two Kids	二 竖	Diseases
Homophonic substitution	通 假	Interchangeable and borrowed usage of Chinese characters
Taboo substitution	避 讳	Names of emperors or elders not being used directly either in writing or in speech
Zhen Quan	甄 权	An acupuncturist in the Tang Dynasty

(2) Fundamentals of T.C.M.

Term	Synonym	Chinese
Yuan-source qi	• Yuan qi • Primary qi • Primordial qi	原 气
	Original qi	元 气
Gao	Diaphragm	膏(鬲)
Huang	Omentum	肓

(3) Meridians and points

Term	Synonym	Chinese
Yuan-source points	Yuan-primordial points	原 穴
Luo-connecting points		络 穴
Xi-cleft points		郄 穴

(4) Chapters of *The Inner Classic*

The Spiritual Pivot

Term	Synonym	Chinese
Division of One Day into Four Seasons Conforming to Qi	*Shun Qi Yi Ri Fen Wei Si Shi*	顺气一日分为四时

(5) Issues of *The Classic of Questioning*

Term	Pinyin & Chinese	Main Contents
The 62nd Issue	*Liu Shi Er Nan* 六十二难	Yuan-source points
The 66th Issue	*Liu Shi Liu Nan* 六十六难	Yuan-source points

Topic 6

The Confluent Points of the Eight Extraordinary Vessels

1. General knowledge of the confluent points of the eight extraordinary vessels

The confluent points of the eight extraordinary vessels, also known as the "eight confluent points", "eight meridian-intersecting points", "eight ebb-flow points" or "eight points of the eight vessels", are the eight acupoints where the qi of the regular meridians intersects with that of the eight extraordinary vessels. These points are all located below the elbow and knee joints of the four limbs. Their names, meridian associations, and related eight extraordinary vessels are listed in the following table. (Table 1–6)

Table 1–6 The confluent points of the eight extraordinary vessels

Meridian Association	Confluent Points	Related Extraordinary Vessels
Foot Taiyin	Gongsun (SP4)	Thoroughfare vessel
Hand Jueyin	Neiguan (PC6)	Yin link vessel
Hand Shaoyang	Waiguan (TE5)	Yang link vessel
Foot Shaoyang	Zulinqi (GB41)	Belt vessel
Hand Taiyang	Houxi (SI3)	Governor vessel
Foot Taiyang	Shenmai (BL62)	Yang heel vessel
Hand Taiyin	Lieque (LU7)	Conception vessel
Foot Shaoyin	Zhaohai (KI6)	Yin heel vessel

2. The development of the confluent points of the eight extraordinary vessels

2.1 The eight points in *The Inner Classic* and other early works

2.1.1 *The Inner Classic*

> *Discussion on Points* of *The Spiritual Pivot*: (Linqi (GB41)), located in the depression 1.5 *cun* posterior to Xiaxi (GB43), is the Shu-stream point... (Houxi (SI3)), found posterior to the metacarpophalangeal joint on the ulnar side of the hand, is also a Shu-stream point.
>
> *The Meridians* of *The Spiritual Pivot*: The collateral of the hand Taiyin is called Lieque (LU7)... The collateral of the hand heart master is called Neiguan (PC6)... The collateral of the hand Shaoyang is called Waiguan (TE5)... The collateral of the foot Taiyin is called Gongsun (SP4)...
>
> *Discussion on the Cave of Qi* of *Basic Questions*: Four points of the yin and yang heels.
>
> *Discussion on the Mansion of Qi* of *Basic Questions*: One for each of the yin and yang heels.

Gongsun (SP4), Neiguan (PC6), Waiguan (TE5), and Lieque (LU7) are recorded in *The Meridians* of *The Spiritual Pivot*. They are the collaterals of the foot Taiyin, hand Jueyin, hand Shaoyang, and hand Taiyin meridians, respectively.

Houxi (SI3) and Zulinqi (GB41) are recorded in *Discussion on Points* of *The Spiritual Pivot*. Both are Shu-stream points among the five transport points, located on the hand Taiyang and the foot Shaoyang, respectively.

The names Shenmai (BL62) and Zhaohai (KI6) are not mentioned in *The Inner Classic*. However, in *Discussion on the Cave of Qi* and *Discussion on the Mansion of Qi* of *Basic Questions*, there're references to the "four points of the yin and yang heels"; and "one for each of the yin and yang heels". These terms are likely referring to Shenmai (BL62) and Zhaohai (KI6).

2.1.2 *The Systematic Classic of Acupuncture and Moxibustion*

> *Volume 3*: Lieque (LU7), the collateral of the hand Taiyin, diverges towards the Yangming from the point 1.5 *cun* posterior to the wrist...
>
> Neiguan (PC6), the collateral of the hand heart master, diverges towards the Shaoyang from the point 2 *cun* posterior to the palm...

Waiguan (TE5), the collateral of the hand Shaoyang, diverges towards the heart from the depression 2 *cun* posterior to the wrist...

Houxi (SI3), attributed to wood, is located in the depression posterior to the metacarpophalangeal joint on the ulnar side of the little finger of the hand. It's the point where the hand Taiyang meridian infuses, and it is the Shu-stream point...

Gongsun (SP4) diverges towards the Yangming from the point 1 *cun* posterior to the metatarsophalangeal joint of the big toe of the foot, and it's the collateral of the Taiyin...

Zhaohai (KI6), stemming from the yin heel vessel, is located 1 *cun* inferior to the medial malleolus of the foot...

Linqi (GB41), attributed to wood, is located in the depression posterior to the metatarsophalangeal joint of the fourth toe of the foot, and is 1.5 *cun* from Xiaxi (GB43). It's where the foot shaoyang meridian infuses and is the Shu-stream point...

Shenmai (BL62), stemming from the yang heel vessel, is located in the depression inferior to the lateral malleolus of the foot and is approximately the size of a nail...

The third volume of *The Systematic Classic of Acupuncture and Moxibustion*, derived from *The Therapeutic Importance of Acupuncture Points of Bright Hall*, contains records such as the meridian association, location, and properties of the eight points.

2.2 *A Guide to Acupuncture Classics* (*Zhēn Jīng Zhǐ Nán*, 针经指南) and the eight meridian-intersecting points

2.2.1 The origin of the eight meridian-intersecting points

The Preface to the Eight Ebb-Flow Points (*Liú Zhù Bā Xué Xù*, 流注八穴序): The theory of the eight meridian-intersecting points holds the key to acupuncture theories. However, the original author remains unknown, and the only information available is from the preface, which states that this theory originated from the Hermit of Shaoshi Mountain. Recently, its clinical effects have become increasingly evident. When I was young, I obtained a copy from a hermit named Song Zihua, who had practised this theory in the region between the Yellow River and the Huai River for forty-one years. The number of serious patients he successfully treated and the cases that responded quickly to his treatment are beyond count! I immersed myself in this technique to such an extent that only Bolun's addiction to alcohol could compare! However, it's a regret that just as I began to learn it and hadn't yet mastered the fundamentals and skills, a series of wars broke out, causing me to lose all my family's collection of illustrations and the original book as well. It has been 15 years since then, during which I've earnestly searched for the book without success. Recently, I acquired a copy from the Wang family in Beizi, Tongtai. This version is as almost identical to my old collection, except for one or two incorrect characters. However, after studying it, I believe these minor errors will not pose any significant issues.... If the practitioner can make a clear diagnosis and treat the disease using points from both the upper and lower parts of the body (based on the eight meridian-intersecting points), it will be akin to deploying a regular army to capture villains and thieves; the chance of their escape is rare...

As a type of acupoint, the term "eight meridian-intersecting points" was first recorded in *A Guide to Acupuncture Classics* written by Dou Mo during the Jin and Yuan dynasties. While it is referred to as "the eight ebb-flow points" in the text, it is called "the eight meridian-intersecting points" in the preface. From the preface, the method originated from a "hermit of the Shaoshi Mountain", and practitioners of this method found it effective. A hermit named Song Zihua passed this method on to Dou Mou, meaning that Dou Mo was not the originator of the eight meridian-intersecting points. This method had likely been in circulation for some time before Dou Mo.

KNOWLEDGE DATABASE: LITERATURE

A Guide to Acupuncture Classics (*Zhēn Jīng Zhǐ Nán*, 针经指南)

A Guide to Acupuncture Classics was published in 1295 during the Yuan Dynasty. It's a compilation of Dou Mo's works on acupuncture. The most famous article in this book is likely *A Verse to Elucidate Mysteries* (*Biāo Yōu Fù*, 标幽赋).

Dou Mo (1196–1280) was an acupuncturist in his early years before later becoming a high-ranking official. His original name was Dou Jie, with the courtesy name Hanqing. Dou Mo was his later name, and his corresponding courtesy name was Zisheng. Posthumously, he was honored with the official title of Taishi (太师). In the history of acupuncture, Dou Mo may be referred to by any of these names.

KNOWLEDGE DATABASE: PEOPLE

Liu Lin (刘伶)

Liu Ling (刘伶) (c. 221–c. 300), with the courtesy name Bolun (伯伦), was a renowned literary figure in the Jin Dynasty. He was best known for his heavy drinking and disregard for social conventions. It's recorded that he often rode in a cart while drinking and had someone follow him carrying a shovel, with instructions to "bury me where I die".

2.2.2 The confluence of eight points and the indications of eight points

The Confluence of Eight Points (*Bā Xué Jiāo Huì*, 八穴交会) (according to *Formulas for Universal Relief* (*Pǔ Jì Fāng*, 普济方)

Gongsun (SP4), which communicates with the thoroughfare vessel, and Neiguan (PC6), which communicates with the yin link vessel, converge at the chest, heart, and stomach.

Zulinqi (GB41), which communicates with the belt vessel, and Waiguan (TE5), which communicates with the yang link vessel, converge at the outer canthus, retroauricular area, cheek, neck, shoulder, supraclavicular fossa, chest and diaphragm.

Houxi (SI3), which communicates with the governor vessel, and Shenmai (BL62), which communicates with the yang heel vessel, converge at the inner canthus, nape of the neck, ear, shoulder, small intestine, and bladder.

Lieque (LU7), which communicates with the conception vessel, and Zhaohai (KI6), which communicates with the yin heel vessel, converge at the lung system, throat, chest, and diaphragm.

The eight meridian-intersecting points are interconnected through convergence. Considering the indications of these eight points, their convergence refers to the range of indications associated with the corresponding points.

Among the eight points, only Neiguan (PC6) and Waiguan (TE5) are considered to be "independently converged". The remaining six points all converge with other points: Gongsun (SP4) converges with Neiguan (PC6), Zulinqi (GB41) converges with Waiguan (TE5), Houxi (SI3) converges with Shenmai (BL62), Shenmai (BL62) converges with Houxi (SI3), Zhaohai (KI6) converges with Lieque (LU7), and Lieque (LU7) converges with Zhaohai (KI6). All these points have their own indications. When being treated, except for Neiguan (PC6) and Waiguan (TE5), whose indications can be treated independently with their related points, the indications of the other six points should be addressed according to the following principle: "The acupoint directly related to the disease should be needled first according to its location... If the disease is not cured, use its converged point". (Table 1–7)

Table 1–7 Indications and therapeutic methods for the eight meridian-intersecting points

<table>
<tr><th colspan="2">Eight Meridian-Intersecting Points</th><th>SP4</th><th>PC6</th><th>GB41</th><th>TE5</th><th>SI3</th><th>BL62</th><th>LU7</th><th>KI6</th></tr>
<tr><td colspan="2">Number of Indications</td><td>27</td><td>25</td><td>25</td><td>27</td><td>24</td><td>25</td><td>31</td><td>29</td></tr>
<tr><td rowspan="2">Therapeutic Methods</td><td>1st step</td><td>SP4</td><td rowspan="2">PC6</td><td>GB41</td><td rowspan="2">TE5</td><td>SI3</td><td>BL62</td><td>LU7</td><td>KI6</td></tr>
<tr><td>2nd step</td><td>PC6</td><td>TE5</td><td>BL62</td><td>SI3</td><td>KI6</td><td>LU7</td></tr>
</table>

KNOWLEDGE DATABASE: LITERATURE

Formulas for Universal Relief (Pǔ Jì Fāng, 普济方 *)*

Formulas for Universal Relief is the largest existing medical prescription book compiled by Zhu Su and others during the early Ming Dynasty. It can be regarded as a comprehensive collection of prescription books written before the 15th century. The book consists of 168 volumes, with each disease and syndrome discussed and addressed through detailed prescriptions. It offers a rich source of information and significant reference value. In addition, more than half of the texts included in this work have since been lost, making it a great contribution to the preservation of ancient documents. The original text of *The Confluence of Eight Points* is a case study that is missing in some versions of *A Guide to Acupuncture Classics* but can be found in *Formulas for Universal Relief.*

2.3 *Basics of Medical Classics* (*Yī Jīng Xiǎo Xué*, 医经小学) and the eight points confluent with regular meridians

Volume 3: Eight Points Confluent with Regular Meridians (*Juàn Sān · Jīng Mài Jiāo Huì Bā Xué*, 卷三·经脉交会八穴):

Gongsun (SP4) connects with the thoroughfare vessel and is used to treat conditions related to the stomach, heart, and chest. Similarly, Neiguan (PC6) connects with the yin link vessel and has the same therapeutic indications.

Zulinqi (GB41) belongs to the gallbladder meridian and connects with the belt vessel, while Waiguan (TE5) connects with the yang link vessel. Together, these points converge at the outer canthus.

Houxi (SI3) connects with the governor vessel and is used to treat conditions of the inner canthus and the neck. These same indications are also relevant for Shenmai (BL62), which communicates with the yang heel vessel.

Lieque (LU7) connects with the conception vessel, while Zhaohai (KI6) communicates with the yin heel vessel. Together, these points are used to treat the lung system, diaphragm, and throat.

Basics of Medical Classics, authored by Liu Chun, a Ming Dynasty physician, was first published in the 21st year of Hongwu era (1388). This comprehensive medical text elaborates on medical theories with a rhythmic and structured language. In volume 3, there is a rhyme known as *Eight Points Confluent with Regular Meridians*, which was claimed to be from *Acupuncture Classic* (*Zhēn Jīng*, 针经) (another name or version of *The Spiritial Pivot*) by Liu Chun. This rhyme designates the eight meridian-intersecting points as "the eight points confluent with regular meridians". This rhyme was reprinted in various works, including *The Complete Compendium of Acupuncture and Moxibustion* (*Zhēn Jiǔ Dà Quán*, 针灸大全), *A Collection of Gems in Acupuncture and Moxibustion*, and *The Great Compendium of Acupuncture and Moxibustion*. The term "eight points confluent with regular meridians" doesn't emphasize the connection between these eight points and the eight extraordinary vessels.

KNOWLEDGE DATABASE: LITERATURE

***Basics of Medical Classics* (*Yī Jīng Xiǎo Xué*, 医经小学)**

Basics of Medical Classics was written by Liu Chun during the Ming Dynasty. This comprehensive 6-volume medical work was first published in 1388. The third volume is dedicated to meridians, covering topics such as the twelve meridians, the intersection of eight meridians and eight points, the flow of meridians, and the distributions of meridians and points throughout the body.

***The Complete Compendium of Acupuncture and Moxibustion* (*Zhēn Jiǔ Dà Quán*, 针灸大全)**

The Complete Compendium of Acupuncture and Moxibustion, also known as *Quick Methods of Acupuncture and Moxibustion* (*Zhēn Jiǔ Jié Fǎ*, 针灸捷法) or *The Complete Compendium of Quick Methods of Acupuncture and Moxibustion* (*Zhēn Jiǔ Jié Fǎ Dà Quán*, 针灸捷法大全), was written by Xu Feng around 1439 during the Ming Dynasty. This six-volume comprehensive work on acupuncture has had a significant influence, mainly collecting acupuncture rhymes from various schools.

2.4 *The Complete Compendium of Acupuncture and Moxibustion* and the confluent points of the eight extraordinary vessels

The title of the fourth volume of *The Complete Compendium of Acupuncture and Moxibustion* is "*Dou Wen Zhen's Eight Methods of Ebb-Flow* (*Dòu Wén Zhēn Gōng Bā Fǎ Liú Zhù*, 窦文真公八法流注)". This volume includes several rhymes and verses related to the eight points. For example, Liu Chun's *The Eight Points Confluent with Regular Meridians* was renamed *A Rhyme of The Eight Points Confluent with Eight Vessels* (*Bā Mài Jiāo Huì Bā Xué Gē*, 八脉交会八穴歌). The term "the confluent points of eight extraordinary vessels" first appeared here, directly highlighting the relationship between the eight extraordinary vessels and the eight points.

In this volume, there are also *A rhyme of Eight Vessels Matching Eight Diagrams* (*Bā Mài Pèi Bā Guà Gē*, 八脉配八卦歌), *A rhyme of Combination of the Eight Points* (*Bā Xué Xiāng Pèi Hé Gē*, 八穴相配合歌), and *Indications of Eight Methods* (*Bā Fǎ Zhǔ Zhì Bìng Zhèng*, 八法主治病证). Here, the terms "eight vessels", "eight points", and "eight methods" all refer to the confluent points of eight extraordinary vessels.

Indications of Eight Methods is recorded in *The Complete Compendium of Acupuncture and Moxibustion*. However, this article not only compiles the indications for the eight meridian-intersecting points originally from Dou Mo's work but also includes contents copied from other acupuncture and moxibustion texts. As a result, the number of indications it presented was quite different from the actual range of diseases it covered.

Building on the concept of the confluent points of the eight extraordinary vessels and incorporating the theories of the nine palaces and eight diagrams, as well as timely acupuncture and moxibustion, doctors of the Yuan and Ming dynasties developed the "eight methods of flight" and the "eight methods of the sacred tortoise". These methods involved using acupuncture or moxibustion at specific times, utilizing the confluent points of the eight extraordinary vessels. Both methods can be found in *The Complete Compendium of Acupuncture and Moxibustion*. They reflect the understanding of practitioners at that time regarding the influence of time on the body's rhythms. However, since these methods are quite formulaic, they have faced criticism over the years.

2.5 Other works in the Ming and Qing dynasties and the confluent points of the eight extraordinary vessels

After *The Complete Compendium of Acupuncture and Moxibustion*, the confluent points of the eight extraordinary vessels were recorded in various books, including *A Collection of Gems in Acupuncture and Moxibustion*, *Introduction to Medicine* (*Yī Xué Rù Mén*, 医学入门), *The Great Compendium of Acupuncture and Moxibustion*, *Acupuncture Principles in Six Volumes* (*Zhēn Fāng Liù Jí*, 针方六集) and *Golden Mirror of the Medical Tradition*. In these texts, they are also referred to as "the confluent points of the eight extraordinary vessels", "eight points", and "eight methods".

In these books, the combination methods, indications, and their relationships with the extraordinary vessels of the eight confluent points were further elaborated.

KNOWLEDGE DATABASE: LITERATURE

Introduction to Medicine (*Yī Xué Rù Mén*, 医学入门)

Introduction to Medicine was written by Li Chan and published in 1575 during the Ming Dynasty. This comprehensive medical text consists of eight volumes, including an introductory volume titled "Opening Volume". It primarily contains literary compositions in rhymes, which are sometimes called songs, odes, or verses, which are thoroughly annotated by the author. Volume 1 of the book focuses on acupuncture.

Acupuncture Principles in Six Volumes (*Zhēn Fāng Liù Jí*, 针方六集)

Acupuncture Principles in Six Volumes was written by Wu Kun and published in 1618 during the Ming Dynasty. The book is divided into six volumes and introduces the basic theories of acupuncture and moxibustion.

3. Note

The term "eight meridian-intersecting points" lays emphasis on "eight points", whereas in the term "confluent points of the eight extraordinary vessels", the focus appears to be on the "eight extraordinary vessels" as the central aspect of the eight-point theory. In fact, an analysis of the development of the nomenclature for the eight meridian-intersecting points reveals that their significance doesn't lie in the communication between the eight extraordinary vessels and the twelve meridians, but in the methods of point combination and clinical experience they embody. However, since the indications of the eight confluent points cannot be easily explained by the theory of meridian attribution of acupoints, the pathways of the eight extraordinary vessels may be used to provide an explanation.

The eight confluent points include four on the upper limbs and four on the lower limbs. All four points on the upper limbs are located above the wrist, except for Houxi (SI3), and they are generally situated higher. In contrast, the four points on the lower limbs are located below the ankle and are generally positioned lower. The locations and meridians of the upper and lower points in each pair generally correspond: Lieque (LU7) and Zhaohai (KI6) are both located near the wrist or ankle joint, Houxi (SI3) and Shenmai (BL62) both belong to the Taiyang meridians, and Zulinqi (GB41) and Waiguan (TE5) both belong to the Shaoyang meridians. Additionally, Gongsun (SP4) and Neiguan (PC6) are both situated in the middle of the medial aspect of the upper or lower limb. The four pairs of points, with corresponding locations and similar therapeutic effects, can achieve the function of "treating the disease using points from both the upper and lower parts of the body". This forms the foundation for applying the eight meridian-intersecting points in upper-lower combinations.

Inspired by the eight confluent points, practitioners in later periods expanded the combination and application of acupoints. The *four gate* (Sì Guān, 四关) point combination, which includes Hegu (LI4) and Taichong (LR3) and was proposed in modern times, aligns with the combination pattern of the eight confluent points.

Reflections

Can the eight confluent points be used to treat various diseases throughout the body?

Terms and Synonyms

(1) History, culture and people

Term	Chinese	Explanations
Liu Ling	刘 伶	A heavy drinker known for his literary reputation during the Jin Dynasty
Dou Mo	窦 默	The author of *A Guide to Acupuncture Classics*

(continued)

Term	Chinese	Explanations
Dou Hanqing	窦汉卿	The author of *A Guide to Acupuncture Classics*
Dou Zisheng	窦子声	
Dou Taishi	窦太师	
Zhu Su	朱 橚	The author of *Formulas for Universal Relief*
Liu Chun	刘 纯	The author of *Basics of Medical Classics*
Xu Feng	徐 凤	The author of *The Complete Compendium of Acupuncture and Moxibustion*
Li Chan	李 梴	The author of *Introduction to Medicine*
Wu Kun	吴 崐	The author of *Acupuncture Principles in Six Volumes*

(2) Meridians and points

Term	Synonym	Chinese
Eight confluent points		八脉交会穴
	Eight meridian-intersecting points	交经八穴
	The confluence of eight points	八穴交会穴
	Eight points confluent with regular meridians	经脉交会八穴

(3) Book names

Term	Synonym	Chinese
A Guide to Acupuncture Classics	*Zhen Jing Zhi Nan*	针经指南
Formulas for Universal Relief	*Pu Ji Fang*	普济方
Basics of Medical Classics	*Yi Jing Xiao Xue*	医经小学
The Complete Compendium of Acupuncture and Moxibustion	*Zhen Jiu Da Quan*	针灸大全
	• *Quick Methods of Acupuncture and Moxibustion* • *Zhen Jiu Jie Fa*	针灸捷法
	• *The Complete Compendium of Quick Methods of Acupuncture and Moxibustion* • *Zhen Jiu Jie Fa Da Quan*	针灸捷法大全

(continued)

Term	Synonym	Chinese
Introduction to Medicine	*Yi Xue Ru Men*	医学入门
Acupuncture Principles in Six Volumes	*Zhen Fang Liu Ji*	针方六集

Chapter 2
Acumox Techniques

Guidance

Understand the evolution of Deqi and the differing historical opinions on reinforcing and reducing techniques in acupuncture.

Be familiar with the development of moxibustion.

Topic 1

Reinforcing and Reducing in Acupuncture Techniques

1. General introduction to the reinforcing and reducing techniques in acupuncture

Nine Needles and Twelve Yuan-Source Points of *The Spiritual Pivot* states: "To apply the needle, the deficient should be reinforced, the full should be discharged, the stagnation should be eliminated, and the predominance of evils should be reduced". It also notes, "The key to reinforcing the deficient and reducing the excessive lie in the use of the nine needles, which are the most effective. The effects of reinforcing and reducing can be achieved through the application of needles." The reinforcing and reducing techniques in acupuncture are based on these elaborations. Along with other discussions in *The Inner Classic*, two types of needling techniques were developed to reinforce the deficient and reduce the excessive. These techniques include various manipulations such as reinforcing and reducing techniques by speed, thrusting and lifting, twisting and rotating, changing direction, coordinating with respiration, and employing opening and closing techniques, among others. Although the concepts of deficiency and excess in the acupuncture principles of *The Inner Classic* primarily refer to the results of pulse diagnosis and should not be equated with the deficiency and excess of diseases or syndromes (**see Topic 12**), later interpretations have generally understood deficiency-reinforcing and excess-reducing needling techniques as addressing two distinct issues: insufficiency and surplus.

In modern acupuncture techniques, needling methods that can restore weakened functions of the body to their normal state referred to as reinforcing techniques, while those that restore the body's excessive functions to their normal state are called reducing techniques. It's generally believed that the effects of reinforcing and reducing techniques in acupuncture are determined by the body's condition at the time, the relative specificity of acupoint actions, and the quality of the acupuncture techniques.

When proposing the use of needles to reinforce the deficient and reduce the excessive, *The Inner Classic* also expressed the view that needles should not be used to treat deficient syndromes. Later, practitioners further explored this notion and argued that "needles cannot reinforce but reduce".

2. The development of "Needles cannot reinforce but reduce"

2.1 *The Inner Classic*

Symptoms and Signs of Zang-fu Organs Caused by Evil Qi of *The Spiritual Pivot* (*Líng Shū · Xié Qì Zàng Fǔ Bìng Xíng*, 灵枢 · 邪气脏腑病形): Huang Di asked: "Regarding the six variations of diseases, what types of acupuncture techniques can be applied?" Qi Bo answered: "... Those small pulses indicate the insufficiency of yin, yang, and physique-qi. Such cases can't be treated with needles but can be regulated with medication that has a sweet flavour."

Origin and Terminal of *The Spiritual Pivot*: Huang Di asked: "What about the normal and adverse effects of physique-qi?" Qi Bo answered: "Insufficient physique-qi and superabundant morbid-qi indicate an excess of evils, which should be reduced immediately. Conversely, superabundant physique-qi with insufficient morbid-qi should be reinforced promptly. If both physique-qi and morbid-qi are insufficient, it indicates insufficiency of both yin and yang, which should not be treated with acupuncture. Needling in this case would worsen the deficiency, leading to a further depletion of yin, yang, blood and qi. Thus, the five zang organs will be depleted, the tendons, bones, and marrow will become dry, the elderly will die, and those in their prime will be unable to recover. Cases with superabundant physique-qi and morbid-qi are referred to as a superabundance of both yin and yang. In such situations, the evil should be reduced instantly to adjust the deficiency and excess. Therefore, it's said that the superabundant should be reduced and the insufficient should be reinforced. This refers to the situation described above."

Ending and Beginning of *The Spiritual Pivot* (*Líng Shū · Zhōng Shǐ*, 灵枢 · 终始): In patients with insufficient qi, both Maikou and Renying are weak and don't correspond to their expected sizes. In these cases, both yin and yang are insufficient. However, if yang is supplemented, yin may become further depleted and if yin is reduced, yang may be diminished. Such conditions can be treated with herbs of a sweet flavour. If this approach is ineffective, more potent medications may be necessary.

The Length of Meridians of *The Spiritual Pivot*: (Minute collaterals) that are excessively full of stagnated blood should be promptly induced to bleed. Excessive conditions should be reduced, while deficient ones should be treated with medication to reinforce them.

Jade Tablets of *The Spiritual Pivot* (*Líng Shū · Yù Bǎn*, 灵 枢 · 玉 版): Qi Bo said: "(The needle) can kill the living but cannot rescue the dead... The source of qi that people receive comes from food. The place where food enters is the stomach. The stomach is considered the sea of water, food, qi, and blood. The movement of clouds from the sea occurs under the sky. Similarly, the transformation of qi and blood from the stomach is carried out through the meridians. The meridians are the major collaterals of the five zang and six fu organs. If they're confronted and deprived, things will go wrong." Huang Di said, "Is there a rule that applies throughout the entire body?" Qi Bo said, "When Wuli (LI13) is confronted, the qi will stagnate during manipulation and may go awry after five stimulations. Performing the procedure five times will deplete the qi of zang organs, and repeating this five times, a total of twenty-five, will exhaust its ability to transfuse qi. This is referred to as 'depriving the natural qi', which doesn't mean causing deaths." Huang Di said, "I'd like to understand it in more detail." Qi Bo said: "If someone is observed and then attacked at the door, they will die in the inner room; if someone is attacked while inside the door, they will die in the lobby."

Symptoms and Signs of Zang-fu Organs Caused by Evil Qi of *The Spiritual Pivot* and *Ending and Beginning* of *The Spiritual Pivot* both state that if the pulse diagnosis reveals a deficiency in yin, yang, and physique-qi, the condition can't be treated with needles but rather with medications that has a sweet flavour. In *Origin and Terminal* of *The Spiritual Pivot*, the concepts of constitution (physique-qi) and disease (morbid-qi) are compared. If both the constitution and the disease show signs of deficiency, it indicates a deficiency of both yin and yang, and such a condition can't be treated with needles. *The Length of Meridians* of *The Spiritual Pivot* also states that in cases of deficiency, the minute collaterals should be treated with medication. According to these texts, needles are contraindicated for treating deficient syndromes characterized by insufficient yin, yang, and physique-qi. This forms the basis for the later saying that "needles cannot reinforce but reduce".

Jade Tablets of *The Spiritual Pivot* states that the needle "can kill the living but cannot rescue the dead". This is because the meridians are the major collaterals for qi and blood to flow through the five zang organs and six fu organs. If acupuncture prohibitions are violated, such as needling points like Wuli (LI13), the consequence can be "depriving the natural qi". This may result in "depleting the qi of zang organs" or even "exhausting its ability to transfuse qi". In other words, "if they're being confronted and deprived, things will go wrong". This also suggests from another perspective that, regarding the qi and blood in the human body, needles can only have a reducing effect and not a reinforcing effect.

KNOWLEDGE DATABASE: LITERATURE

Symptoms and Signs of Zang-fu Organs Caused by Evil Qi of *The Spiritual Pivot* (*Líng Shū · Xié Qì Zàng Fǔ Bìng Xíng*, 灵枢 · 邪气脏腑病形): The 4th chapter of the *Ling Shu*. It primarily discusses the manifestations of evil qi attacking the body.

Ending and Beginning of *The Spiritual Pivot* (*Líng Shū · Zhōng Shǐ*, 灵枢 · 终始): The 9th chapter of the *Ling Shu*. It mainly focuses on the fundamentals of acupuncture, including techniques for reinforcing and reducing, needling depth, diagnosis, therapeutic principles, and point selection.

Jade Tablets of *The Spiritual Pivot* (*Líng Shū · Yù Bǎn*, 灵枢 · 玉版): The 60th chapter of the *Ling Shu*. This chapter emphasizes the importance of prevention, diagnosis, and early-stage treatment, using carbuncles and abscesses as examples.

2.2 *Teachings of [Zhu] Danxi* (*Dān Xī Xīn Fǎ*, 丹溪心法)

> *Miscellaneous Discussions on Overlooked Pieces* (*Shí Yí Zá Lùn*, 拾遗杂论): The needling techniques are solely for reducing and not reinforcing.

Zhu Zhenheng, a physician of the Yuan Dynasty, stated that "the needling techniques are solely for reducing and not reinforcing", but he didn't provide an explanation for his view.

KNOWLEDGE DATABASE: LITERATURE

Teachings of [Zhu] Danxi (*Dān Xī Xīn Fǎ*, 丹溪心法)

The term "Zhu" in the book title "*Teachings of [Zhu] Danxi*" indicates the surname of Danxi. Zhu Danxi refers to the physician Zhu Zhenheng from the Yuan Dynasty. This book is a collection of Zhu Danxi's experiences, opinions, and comments on medicine, recorded and compiled by his students. Although Zhu Danxi lived during the Yuan Dynasty, this book was published in 1481 during the Ming Dynasty. It's a comprehensive medical text.

Danxi is neither a name nor a courtesy name. Zhu Zhenheng's courtesy name was Yanxiu. The term Danxi literally means "red brook", referring to the area where Zhu Zhenheng lived. In Chinese tradition, a respected person can also be referred to by the name of their hometown. Therefore, "Danxi" was used as a respectful title for Zhu Zhenheng by others.

2.3 *Correct Instructions of Medicine* (*Yī Xué Zhèng Chuán*, 医学正传)

> *Volume 1: Possible Questions on Medicine* (*Juàn Yī · Yī Xué Huò Wèn*, 卷一 · 医学或问):

Although it's said that there are techniques for reinforcing and reducing with needles, I'm afraid that needles cannot reinforce but reduce. *The Inner Classic* states that reducing involves "reducing by confronting", where the needle confronts the incoming qi of the meridian and lets it out, thereby reducing the excess. Conversely, reinforcing is described as "reinforcing by following", where the needle follows the departing qi to retain it, but this does not necessarily tonify the deficiency. Or else, why are there sayings in *The Inner Classic* as: "Do not needle exuberant heat, do not needle disorderly pulses, and do not needle profuse sweating", and "do not needle people with extreme fatigue, do not needle people with great hunger, do not needle people with excessive thirst, do not needle people who have just eaten, and do not needle people who're severely frightened"? Additionally, there're sayings such as: "if both physique-qi and morbid-qi are insufficient, it indicates insufficiency of both yin and yang, which should not be treated with acupuncture. Needling in this case would worsen the deficiency, leading to a further depletion of qi. Thus, the elderly will die, and those in their prime will be unable to recover." All these texts discuss reducing without reinforcing. Those who're learning must understand this.

Correct Instructions of Medicine, written by Yu Tuan, a Ming Dynasty physician, primarily adopted Zhu Zhenheng's theories and also integrated views from other practitioners to elaborate his own perspective. In the opening chapter, *Possible Questions on Medicine*, Yu Tuan inherited Zhu Zhenheng's view that "the needling techniques are solely for reducing and not reinforcing". He proposed that "needles cannot reinforce but reduce", and provided examples of acupuncture contraindications from *The Inner Classic* to support this stance.

KNOWLEDGE DATABASE: LITERATURE

Correct Instructions of Medicine (*Yī Xué Zhèng Chuán*, 医学正传)

Correct Instructions of Medicine was compiled by Yu Tuan in 1515 during the Ming Dynasty, who greatly valued Zhu Danxi's medical theories. Yu Tuan observed numerous misunderstandings about medicine at that time, which motivated him to compile the book to represent correct and well-established theories. As a result, the book is sometimes translated as *Orthodox Transmission of Medicine*.

The pinyin of this book is sometimes written as *Yī Xué Zhèng Zhuàn*. This results from a misunderstanding of the character "传", which has two pronunciations: zhuàn and chuán. They have different meanings: zhuàn means biography, while chuán means to pass on, to teach, or something inherited. From the preface of the book, it's clear that the author intended not to write a historical account but to introduce correct theories. Therefore, the character "传" should be read as chuán and written as chuán in pinyin of the book's title.

2.4 *Questions and Answers on Acupuncture and Moxibustion* (*Zhēn Jiǔ Wèn Duì*, 针灸问对)

Volume 1: ...From this, it can be inferred that the indications for nine needles are primarily due to the invasion of external evils. The reducing by needles specifically addresses the disease condition. Nowadays, if people have such diseases, acupuncture should definitely be used. However, if the pathogenic factors are excessive and the original qi has already been weakened, acupuncture will be of no help. For example, in the case of yin deficiency and hyperactivity of fire in consumptive diseases, the therapeutic principles should focus on nourishing yin and reducing fire. However, can acupuncture effectively nourish yin? In the case of lung heat causing burned lobes in *Wei* syndromes, the therapeutic principles should involve clearing the lung and supplementing water. However, can acupuncture effectively supplement water? This is what the saying in *The Inner Classic* means: "...Insufficiency of yin, yang, and physique-qi, such cases can't be treated with needles but can be regulated with medication that has a sweet flavour". When we understand this, we can determine whether a condition is suitable for acupuncture treatment. However, what should those majoring in acupuncture do if they lack skills in pulse diagnosis and body observation? They might simply ask about the problem and then needle some points directly. It's natural that this approach can lead to stubborn cases resulting from improper needle techniques. Though this approach may occasionally yield positive results, it's often just by chance. Some practitioners may boast about their remarkable needling techniques, but won't such claims be ridiculed by those who know their mistakes?

Volume 2: *The Inner Classic* states: Insufficient yang can be warmed with qi, and insufficient yin can be nourished with flavours. However, needles are made of stone, which contains neither qi nor flavour. What's more, it injures the skin and flesh and creates a hole in the body. Qi escapes through this hole, so how can this process be considered reinforcing? ... To reinforce this, the principle of "circle" should be employed. "Circle" signifies movement and movement implies changing location. This approach helps disperse stagnant qi and promote circulation as well as transform an unresolved pulse and aid in its recovery. Reducing involves alleviating excess, while reinforcing is about dispersing stagnated qi and transforming an unresolved pulse. Doesn't "dispersing" and "changing" refer to reducing? Moreover, if we examine the application of the nine needles described in the *Basic Questions*, all of them are classified as reducing techniques. Danxi wouldn't speak without basis. Reinforcing techniques are indeed mentioned in *The Inner Classic*, and it's just what Mr. Zhang expressed in his saying that "to remove evils is actually to support the vital qi, to remove the old is actually to generate the new".

Wang Ji, a Ming Dynasty physician, adhered to Zhu Danxi and Yu Tuan's view that "needles cannot reinforce but reduce". In the first volume of *Questions and Answers on Acupuncture and Moxibustion*, he examined the materials and functions of the nine needles and believed that they were used primarily for treating diseases caused by external pathogens. The so-called reinforcing techniques in acupuncture are actually another way of expressing Zhang Zihe's view that "to remove evils is actually to support the vital qi, to remove the old is actually to generate the new".

These opinions and discussions of Wang Ji were later compiled in *The Great Compendium of Acupuncture and Moxibustion* (*Zhēn Jiǔ Dà Chéng*, 针灸大成).

KNOWLEDGE DATABASE: LITERATURE

***Questions and Answers on Acupuncture and Moxibustion* (*Zhēn Jiǔ Wèn Duì*, 针灸问对)**

This book is sometimes referred to as "针灸问答" (*Zhēn Jiǔ Wèn Dá*). In this context, "对" and "答" both mean "answer".

The book was compiled in 1530 by Wang Ji, who was primarily a physician but also had a keen interest in acupuncture. While studying acupuncture, he began to question whether contemporary doctors adhered to the guidelines of *The Inner Classic* and *The Classic of Questioning*. This led him to compile the book as a review of various techniques, theories, and treatments related to acupuncture and moxibustion.

KNOWLEDGE DATABASE: PEOPLE

Zhang Zihe (张子和)

In the selected text, "Mr. Zhang" refers to Zhang Congzhen (张从正) (c. 1156–1228), renowned for his theory of eliminating evils. His courtesy name was "Zihe (子和)" , and he also had the literary name "Dairen (戴人)".

2.5 *Introduction to Medicine*

Volume 1: Acupuncture and Moxibustion (*Juàn Yī · Zhēn Jiǔ*, 卷一 · 针灸): Moxibustion: ... Although it's said that there're techniques for reinforcing and reducing with the needles, I'm afraid that they can cannot reinforce but reduce... Conditions such as deficiency, impairment, critical illnesses, and prolonged diseases are all unsuitable for needle treatment.

Li Chan, a Ming Dynasty physician, referenced Yu Tuan's discussion in his *Introduction to Medicine*, noting that "needles cannot reinforce but reduce". He argued that needles were unsuitable for treating conditions of deficiency and impairment, as well as critical and chronic diseases. Liao Runhong, a physician of the Qing Dynasty, incorporated this view into his *Grand Compendium of Acupuncture and Moxibustion* (*Zhēn Jiǔ Jí Chéng*, 针灸集成).

KNOWLEDGE DATABASE: LITERATURE

***Grand Compendium of Acupuncture and Moxibustion* (*Zhēn Jiǔ Jí Chéng*, 针灸集成)**

Grand Compendium of Acupuncture and Moxibustion, written by Liao Runhong (1835–?), was published in 1874 during the Qing Dynasty. In this four-volume work, the author referenced ancient literature on acupuncture and moxibustion and offered his own insights, such as research on acupoints.

2.6 *The Classified Classic*

Volume 16: Needling Nue[1] *of Various Meridians* (*Juàn Shí Liù · Zhū Jīng Nuè Cì*, 卷十六 · 诸经疟刺): If the Nue pulse is slow, large, and weak, medication should be used accordingly, and needles are not suitable. Needles cannot reinforce but reduce, making them unsuitable for patients with weak pulses. In the chapter *The Length of Meridians*, it's stated that "excessive conditions should be reduced, while deficient ones should be treated with medication to reinforce them", and this is just one example.

Volume 22: The High, the Low, the Adverse, and the Normal (*Juàn Èr Shí Èr · Guì Jiàn Nì Shùn*, 卷二十二 · 贵贱逆顺): If both physique-qi and morbid-qi are insufficient, it indicates insufficiency of both yin and yang, which should not be treated with acupuncture. Needling in this case would worsen the deficiency, leading to a further depletion of yin, yang, blood and qi. Thus, the five zang organs will be depleted, the tendons, bones, and marrow will become dry, the elderly will die, and those in their prime will be unable to recover. Yang governs the exterior, while yin governs the interior. If both the physique-qi and the morbid-qi are insufficient, it indicates a deficiency of both exterior and interior yin and yang. This condition is least suitable for acupuncture treatment. If acupuncture is still used in this situation, it will further weaken the deficiency, leading to the exhaustion of blood and qi and causing the tendons and marrows to dry out. The elders will become more exhausted and may die as a result, while those in their prime will become debilitated and unable to recover to their original conditions. Cases

1. Nue: The pinyin translation for " 疟 ", which originally means "alternating chills and fever". While it's sometimes translated as malaria, this is not entirely accurate.

with superabundant physique-qi and morbid-qi are referred to as a superabundance of both yin and yang. In such situations, the evil should be reduced instantly to adjust the deficiency and excess. The superabundance of both physique-qi and morbid-qi indicates an excess of pathogenic factors, so immediate reduction techniques should be applied. Therefore, it is clear that this is an excessive condition. Why is it important to adjust the deficiency and excess? This is because before needling, we must prepare for the potential of a false-excess condition; after needling, we must prevent sudden deficiency. Therefore, adjustment is necessary. Therefore, it's said that the superabundant should be reduced and the insufficient should be reinforced. This refers to the situation described above. To apply the needle, the deficient should be reinforced, the full should be discharged. Thus, it's said that "the key to reinforcing the deficient and reducing the excessive lie in the use of the nine needles, which are the most effective. The effects of reinforcing and reducing can be achieved through the application of needles." One might ask that using reinforcing techniques for deficient cases means that the condition of weak Cunkou should be reinforced, and using discharging techniques for full cases means that the condition of excessive Cunkou should be reduced. This is the general principle of acupuncture, where it seems that all deficiencies can be reinforced. However, the texts mention that "if both physique-qi and morbid-qi are insufficient, it indicates insufficiency of both yin and yang, which should not be treated with acupuncture". Why is this the case? *Discussion on Treasuring Life and Preserving Physique* (*Bǎo Mìng Quán Xíng Lùn*, 宝命全形论) states that "There're both deficiency and excess in humans. Avoid approaching the five types of deficiency, but do not be distant from the five types of excess". *Five Exterior Manifestations and Five Emissaries* (*Wǔ Yuè Wǔ Shǐ*, 五阅五使) notes that "when blood and qi are abundant, and the muscles are hard and tight, needles can be applied". *Discussion on Strange Diseases* (*Qí Bìng Lùn*, 奇病论) states that "the advice to avoid impairing the deficient means not to use chan-needles or bian-stones for emaciation". *Discussion on Shen* (*Běn Shén*, 本神) advises that "acupuncture practitioners should observe the patient's posture to determine whether the spirit and soul have survived or perished. If the five zang organs are impaired, needles shouldn't be used." *Explanations of the Small Needle* (*Xiǎo Zhēn Jiě*, 小针解) states that "the notion that death results from selecting the vessels of five zang organs means that the disease is central and the qi is insufficient, but needles are used to completely and drastically discharge all yin vessels". *The Length of Meridians* mentions that "excessive conditions should be reduced, while deficient ones should be treated with medication to reinforce them". *Symptoms and Signs of Zang-fu Organs Caused by Evil Qi* states that "Those small pulses indicate the insufficiency of yin, yang, and physique-qi. Such cases can't be treated with needles but can be regulated with medication that has a sweet flavour". All these excerpts emphasize that deficiencies can't be treated with needling. Upon reviewing all the chapters of this classic text, it becomes evident that diseases requiring needling are primarily due to evils retained in the meridians or collaterals, or qi reversal in the zang-fu organs, and most of these are excessive syndromes. Thus, it's clear that needles are effective for reducing but not for reinforcing. But why does it suggest nourishing the insufficient? This is because blood and qi constantly circulate within the human body, and the meridians flow and circulate continuously. Sometimes nourishing yin can help balance yang, and strengthening one aspect can help address another. All these measures aim to harmonize yin and yang and regulate blood and qi, ensuring that there is no relative excess and thus balance can be achieved. This is the essence of what reinforcing and reducing mean. If someone doesn't understand the reason behind reinforcing deficiencies, and lacks insight into its meaning, they might use needles to adjust and nourish various deficiencies of ying and wei, such as emaciation of the body and appearance, essence deficiency, and qi exhaustion. However, this approach could potentially harm the original qi instead. Thus, there will inevitably be cases of immediate failure. The theory that "needles cannot reinforce but reduce" is highlighted in the discussions throughout these chapters. Acupuncture practitioners should be well aware of this crucial principle.

In *The Classified Classic*, Zhang Jingyue compiled discussions on why deficient syndromes can't be treated with needling as described in *The Inner Classic*. He provided the theoretical basis for the notion that "needles cannot reinforce but reduce". Meanwhile, he analyzed the reinforcing and reducing techniques of acupuncture in *The Inner Classic* from a medical theory perspective and pointed out that the so-called reinforcing and reducing were not intended to treat deficiency syndromes directly, but rather to create a state where "there is no relative excess and thus balance can be achieved".

KNOWLEDGE DATABASE

The Spiritual Pivot (*Líng Shū*, 灵枢)

Five Exterior Manifestations and Five Emissaries (*Wǔ Yuè Wǔ Shǐ*, 五阅五使): The 37th chapter of the *Ling Shu*. It primarily focuses on the observation of external manifestations of the five zang organs.

Discussion on Shen (*Běn Shén*, 本神): The 8th chapter of the *Ling Shu*. It introduces the connotations of various mental activities and emphasizes the significance of shen in acupuncture.

Explanations of the Small Needle (*Xiǎo Zhēn Jiě*, 小针解): The 3rd chapter of the *Ling Shu*. It mainly explains the contents of the *Nine Needles and Twelve Yuan-Source Points*, which are detailed in the first chapter of *The Spiritual Pivot*.

Basic Questions (*Sù Wèn*, 素问)

Discussion on Treasuring Life and Preserving Physique (*Bǎo Mìng Quán Xíng Lùn*, 宝命全形论): The 25th chapter of the *Su Wen*. It argues that to treasure life and preserve physical health, one must understand the relationship between qi and blood in the human body and the changes in nature.

Discussion on Strange Diseases (*Qí Bìng Lùn*, 奇病论): The 47th chapter of the *Su Wen*. It covers the aetiology, clinical manifestations, treatment, and prognosis of various rare and unusual diseases.

3. Note

The statement "Predominance of evil qi indicates excess, while deprived essence qi indicates deficiency" is a common modern interpretation of the concepts of deficiency and excess. However, this does not encompass the full meaning of deficiency and excess as presented in *The Inner Classic*. As the *Discussion on the Separation and Combination of Genuine Qi and Evil Qi* of *Basic Questions* (*Sù Wèn · Lí Hé Zhēn Xié Lùn*, 素问 · 离合真邪论) explains: "*The Classics* state that the excess and deficiency of qi means the shifting and movement between the left and the right. The lower can be regulated from the upper, and the right can be regulated from the left. The concept of surplus and insufficiency can be reinforced or reduced in acupoints such as the Xing-spring and Shu-stream points; this is my understanding. This is due to the shifting and movement of the nutrient qi and the defensive qi, which results in the deficiency and excess of qi and blood, rather than being caused by evil qi entering the meridians from outside." The deficiency and excess mentioned here are caused by the "shifting and movement of the nutrient qi and the defensive qi", which refers to the abnormal distribution of meridian qi. The "excess and deficiency" which "can be reinforced or reduced in acupoints such as the Xing-spring and the Shu-stream", pertain to this condition.

While proposing that "the effects of reinforcing and reducing can be achieved by the application of needles", *The Inner Classic* also notes that needling is not suitable for conditions involving "deficiency of yin, yang, and physique-qi". This reflects the concept that "deprived essence qi indicates deficiency", which is clearly different from the deficiency and excess resulting from the "shifting and movement of the nutrient qi and defensive qi". The indications for acupuncture can be clarified by examining the discussion from later practitioners that "needles cannot reinforce but reduce". In clinical practice, for patients with yin-yang imbalances and dysfunctions resulting from irregular qi activities, the use of reinforcing and reducing techniques can be beneficial. However, for patients with weak constitutions and signs of deficiency syndromes, prioritizing "medication with a sweet flavour" should be considered first.

KNOWLEDGE DATABASE: LITERATURE

Discussion on the Separation and Combination of Genuine Qi and Evil Qi of *Basic Questions* (*Sù Wèn · Lí Hé Zhēn Xié Lùn*, 素问 · 离合真邪论): The 27th chapter of the *Su Wen*. It mainly introduces the different principles for various conditions that arise after evil qi invades the body and interacts with genuine qi.

Reflections

(1) Read the articles on reinforcing and reducing techniques of acupuncture in *The Inner Classic*, and analyze the characteristics of the indications for acupuncture as described in this text.

(2) What are the common diseases treated in an acupuncture clinic? What are the differentiating results of excess and deficiency patterns? Are there any differences between these two types in therapeutic effects?

(3) Can acupuncture be used for individuals with insufficient yin, yang, or physique-qi?

Terms and Synonyms

(1) History, culture and people

Term	Chinese	Explanations
Zhang Congzhen	张从正	A doctor from the Jin (Kin) Dynasty, renowned for his theory on eliminating evils.
Zhang Zihe	张子和	
Zhang Dairen	张戴人	
Zhu Danxi	朱丹溪	A doctor from the Yuan Dynasty, whose experiences, opinions and theories significantly contributed to *Teachings of [Zhu] Danxi*
Zhu Zhenheng	朱震亨	
Yu Tuan	虞　抟	The author of *Correct Instructions of Medicine*
Wang Ji	汪　机	The author of *Questions and Answers on Acupuncture and Moxibustion*
Liao Runhong	廖润鸿	The author of *Grand Compendium of Acupuncture and Moxibustion*

(2) Fundamentals of T.C.M.

Term	Synonym	Chinese
Maikou		脉　口
	Cunkou	寸　口
	Qikou	气　口

(3) Acumox techniques

Term	Synonym	Chinese
Bian-stone	Needling stone	砭 石
Chan-needle	Sagittate needle	镵 针
Twisting	• Twirling • Rotating	捻 转
Reinforcing and reducing	Supplementation and drainage	补 泻

(4) Book names

Term	Synonym	Chinese
Teachings of [Zhu] Danxi	*Dan Xi Xin Fa*	丹溪心法
Correct Instructions of Medicine	• *Orthodox Transmission of Medicine* • *Yi Xue Zheng Chuan* • *Yi Xue Zheng Zhuan* (incorrect)	医学正传
Questions and Answers on Acupuncture and Moxibustion	• *Zhen Jiu Wen Dui*	• 针灸问对
	• *Zhen Jiu Wen Da*	• 针灸问答
Grand Compendium of Acupuncture and Moxibustion	*Zhen Jiu Ji Cheng*	针灸集成

(5) Chapters of *The Inner Classic*

The Spiritual Pivot

Term	Synonym	Chinese
Explanations of the Small Needle	*Xiao Zhen Jie*	小针解
Symptoms and Signs of Zang-fu Organs Caused by Evil Qi	*Xie Qi Zang Fu Bing Xing*	邪气脏腑病形
Discussion on Shen	*Ben Shen*	本 神
Ending and Beginning	*Zhong Shi*	终 始
Five Exterior Manifestations and Five Emissaries	*Wu Yue Wu Shi*	五阅五使
Jade Tablets	*Yu Ban*	玉 版

Basic Questions

Term	Synonym	Chinese
Discussion on Treasuring Life and Preserving Physique	*Bao Ming Quan Xing Lun*	宝命全形论
Discussion on the Separation and Combination of Genuine Qi and Evil Qi	*Li He Zhen Xie Lun*	离合真邪论
Discussion on Strange Diseases	*Qi Bing Lun*	奇病论

Topic 2

Deqi

1. General concepts of Deqi

It's generally believed that Deqi, also known as "arrival of qi", has recently been referred to as the "needling sensation". After the needle is inserted into a certain depth at an acupoint, manipulations such as lifting, thrusting or rotating are performed on the needle. This induces a "meridian qi" response in the needled area, which is referred to as Deqi.

Whether Deqi is achieved can be assessed from two aspects: first, the patient's response to acupuncture, which may include sensations of soreness, distension, heaviness, numbness, and sometimes feelings of heat, cold, pain, twitching, or crawling, as well as sensations that radiate or transmit to specific directions or areas; second, when Deqi is obtained, the practitioner may experience a sinking, tight, or unsmooth feeling while manipulating the needle, or notice the needle body reaction, such as with a quivering sensation.

If Deqi is not induced after needling, the patient won't experience any special sensations or reactions. Meanwhile, the practitioner will have empty, loose, weak, and smooth feelings when manipulating the needle.

2. The development of Deqi

2.1 *The Inner Classic*

Nine Needles and Twelve Yuan-Source Points of *The Spiritual Pivot*: Do not worry about the time if qi doesn't arrive after needling; if qi has been achieved after needling, the needle can be removed and further needling is unnecessary. Needles have different indications based on their shapes, and they should be selected according to their specific functions. The key point of needling is that the effect is achieved upon the arrival of qi. The manifestation of this effect is akin to wind dispersing clouds to reveal a clear sky. This represents the core principle of acupuncture theory.

Explanations of the Small Needle of *The Spiritual Pivot*: The statement that the qi movement in the acupoint is quiet and insensible means that the goal of needling is to achieve Deqi. This requires careful observation to ensure that the optimal timing for needling is not missed.

Ending and Beginning of *The Spiritual Pivot*: The saying that "the effect is achieved upon the arrival of qi" means that excessive conditions will turn deficient by using reducing techniques, and the deficient means that the pulse may be as large as the original but is not as strong as before. If the pulse remains as strong as before, it indicates that the disease has not been cured, even if the patient feels better. When using reinforcing techniques, a deficient condition will turn excessive. Conversely, excessive conditions mean that the pulse may be as large as the original but is stronger. If the pulse is the same as before but not strong, it means the disease has not been cured, even if the patient feels better... All needling methods should aim to achieve Guqi through the use of three-needling techniques... Thus, the first needling is used to expel the yang evil, the second to expel the yin evil; and after the third needling, Guqi will be achieved. The treatment should be concluded upon the arrival of Guqi. The so-called arrival of Guqi means that after the application of reinforcing techniques, the condition becomes excessive, and after the application of reducing techniques, it becomes deficient. This indicates that Guqi has been achieved. When evil qi arrives, it's tight and rapid. In contrast, when Guqi arrives, it's slow and soft... During the application of all needling methods, the body and qi should be observed carefully... The practitioner should focus on shen and pay close attention to the needle. Needles may be inserted shallowly and retained, or inserted slightly and superficially, so as to guide the shen of the patient. Cease the treatment upon the arrival of qi. When yang qi enters the body and yin qi moves outwards, the vital qi can be protected from depletion and the evil qi can be prevented from invading. This condition is referred to as Deqi.

Discussion on the Separation and Combination of Genuine Qi and Evil Qi of *Basic Questions*: ... "Insert the needle while the patient inhales to prevent the reversal of qi. Retain the needle quietly for an extended period to avoid the spread of evil qi. Twist the needle while the patient inhales to achieve Deqi. Remove the needle when the patient exhales and ensure the needle is taken out completely after exhalation. Thus, when the evil qi is expelled, this is referred to as 'reducing'." Huang Di asked: "How do you perform the reinforcing techniques for deficiencies?" Qi Bo replied: "First, palpate the acupoint and move your finger along it. Then, squeeze the acupoint to disperse the qi. Next, push and press the point, and flick the point to ensure the vessel is full. Finally, nail the point and insert the needle. When qi flows smoothly, remove the needle, and simultaneously close the door from the outside to secure the shen. Insert the needle after the patient has completed exhalation, and retain the needle quietly for a prolonged period to facilitate the arrival of qi. As if waiting for a distinguished guest, one should not be concerned about whether it is nightfall. When qi arrives, it should be carefully maintained. Remove the needle when the patient inhales to prevent the qi from escaping. Each needled area should be pressed to close the door to maintain shen qi and preserve the meridian qi. This technique is referred to as reinforcing."

In *The Inner Classic*, there're concepts referred to as the "arrival of qi" and the "arrival of Guqi". According to the explanations in the chapter *Ending and Beginning* in *The Spiritual Pivot* which discusses that "the effect is achieved upon the arrival of qi" and "arrival of Guqi", both are assessed through pulse diagnosis and share the same criteria: excessive conditions will become deficient by using reducing techniques, or it may become excessive after the application of reinforcing techniques. Conversely, deficient conditions will become excessive by using reinforcing techniques, or it may become deficient after the application of reducing techniques. Thus, "arrival of qi" is often used as a shorter form or abbreviation of "arrival of Guqi". In *The Inner Classic*, pulse diagnosis is used to determine whether the "arrival of qi" or "arrival of Guqi" has been achieved, indicating whether acupuncture has been effective.

In *The Inner Classic*, the term "Deqi" is also used. The discussion on reinforcing and reducing techniques often mentions "for the purpose of Deqi" and "for the purpose of the arrival of qi" simultaneously, indicating that they carry the same meaning.

In *The Inner Classic*, the arrival of qi is the ultimate goal of needling techniques. Before achieving the arrival of qi, one should "not worry about the time" and can perform a series of manipulations. These include "insert the needle when the patient inhales", "palpate the acupoint and move your finger along it. Then squeeze the acupoint to disperse the qi. Next, push and press the point, and flick the point to ensure the vessel is full. Finally, nail the point and insert the needle. When qi flows smoothly, remove the needle, and simultaneously close the door from the outside to secure the shen. Insert the needle after the patient has completed exhalation" in order to achieve the arrival of qi. After achieving Deqi, it should be noted that "if qi has been achieved after needling, the needle can be removed and further needling is unnecessary" or "cease the treatment upon the arrival of qi". This means that once qi has arrived, no further treatment is needed, except for the removal of the needle. "Remove the needle when the patient exhales." "Remove the needle when the patient inhales". Such discussions align with the concept that "the effect is achieved upon the arrival of qi". The arrival of qi signifies the effectiveness of acupuncture, and therefore, further stimulation is unnecessary.

2.2 *The Classic of Questioning*

The 70th Issue (*Qī Shí Bā Nàn*, 七十难): In spring and summer, when the weather is warm, the method to induce one yin is as follows: First, insert the needle into the regions of the kidney and liver. After Deqi, withdraw the needle to the superficial layer to induce yin. Autumn and winter are cold seasons. To induce one yang, the method is as follows: First, insert the needle shallowly and superficially into the regions of the heart and lung. After Deqi, push the needle to the deeper layer. This process helps to induce yang.

The 78th Issue (*Qī Shí Bā Nàn*, 七十八难): When performing needling, first use your left hand to press the area to be needled, flick it to make the vessel full, and then nail the area to depress the skin. When the qi manifests as a pulsation in the arteries, the needle can be inserted. After achieving Deqi, push the needle into the deeper layer, which is referred to as reinforcing. Conversely, shaking and lifting the needle into the superficial layer is referred to as reducing. If Deqi cannot be achieved, apply techniques according to the patient's sex and the location of the disease. Without obtaining Deqi, it's impossible to cure the condition.

The Classic of Questioning does not explicitly define the meaning of Deqi, but according to the descriptions provided in this book, the concept of Deqi in *The Classic of Questioning* differs from that presented in *The Inner Classic*. Both the 70th and 78th Issues mention Deqi. However, after achieving Deqi, further manipulations are required in both cases: either pulling up, shaking and lifting the needle into the superficial layer, or pushing the needle into the deep layer. These manipulations are performed to achieve the goals of reinforcing, reducing or tonifying yin or yang.

The Classic of Questioning also highlights the significance of Deqi for prognosis: If Deqi can't be obtained, it's impossible to cure the disease.

KNOWLEDGE DATABASE: LITERATURE

The 70th Issue of *The Classic of Questioning* (*Nàn Jīng · Qī Shí Nàn*, 难经·七十难): The 70th issue of *The Classic of Questioning*. It explains various needling techniques suitable for different seasons.

The 78th Issue of *The Classic of Questioning* (*Nàn Jīng · Qī Shí Bā Nàn*, 难经·七十八难): The 78th issue of *The Classic of Questioning*. It mainly explains the roles of the two hands in needling and the methods for reinforcing and reducing.

2.3 Grand Simplicity of "Huangdi's Inner Classic"

> *Volume 22: Three Needling* (*Juàn Èr Shí Èr · Sān Cì*, 卷二十二 · 三刺): When evil qi arrives, it's tight and rapid. In contrast, when Guqi arrives, it's slow and soft. If the Deqi beneath the needle feels hard and rapid, it indicates the presence of evil qi; if it's slow and soft, it signifies Guqi.

In the chapter *Ending and Beginning* of *The Spiritual Pivot*, it is described that "when evil qi arrives, it's tight and rapid. In contrast, when Guqi arrives, it's slow and soft". From its context, "tight and rapid" and "slow and soft" likely refer to the pulse. Specifically, when evil qi arrives, the pulse will be hard, tight, and rapid. In contrast, when Guqi arrives, the pulse is slow, moderate, and soft.

Yang Shangshan's annotation to this sentence in *Grand Simplicity of "Huangdi's Inner Classic"* can be understood from another viewpoint. He believed that this description pertains to the sensation felt by the practitioner's hand. According to his view, a tight and rapid sensation beneath the needle indicates evil qi, while a slow and soft sensation beneath the needle signifies vital qi.

2.4 Formulas from Benevolent Sages Compiled during the Taiping Era (*Tài Píng Shèng Huì Fāng*, 太平圣惠方)

> *Volume 99* (*Juàn Jiǔ Shí Jiǔ*, 卷九十九): ... Deqi is achieved when the needle reaches the disease, much like a fish taking the bait, which signifies capturing the disease qi. Assess the severity of the condition and treat it according to the meridian. The term "rapid-slow" refers to the process of reaching the disease, which constitutes Deqi.

In the 99th volume of *Formulas from Benevolent Sages Compiled during the Taiping Era*, when explaining that "the deficient is achieved by slow and then rapid manipulation, while the excessive is achieved by rapid and then slow manipulation", it notes that the manifestation of Deqi occurs when the needle is inserted into the body and reaches the location of the disease. This is likened to "a fish taking the bait", with the mechanism being "to capture the disease qi". After this paragraph, there's also the statement "reaching the disease is Deqi". However, the statement is difficult to understand, possibly due to missing texts that follow, which leaves the meaning of this sentence unclear. From the previous text, "Deqi" here is not the same as "Deqi" or "arrival of qi" in *The Inner Classic*. Here, qi specifically refers to "disease qi". However, its manifestation is similar to the concept of Deqi described in *A Verse to Elucidate Mysteries* (*Biāo Yōu Fù*, 标幽赋) (see below) from the Yuan Dynasty.

KNOWLEDGE DATABASE: LITERATURE

Formulas from Benevolent Sages Compiled during the Taiping Era (*Tài Píng Shèng Huì Fāng*, 太平圣惠方)

Formulas from Benevolent Sages Compiled during the Taiping Era was compiled by a group of medical officials led by Wang Huaiyin and organized by the government during the Song Dynasty. This comprehensive 100-volume medical work was published in 992. *Volume 99* of the book is titled "The Classic of Acupuncture", and *Volume 100* is titled "The Bright Hall" which contains "*The Classic of Moxibustion from the Bright Hall*" and "*The Classic of Moxibustion from the Bright Hall for Children*".

2.5 *A Guide to Acupuncture Classics*

A Verse to Elucidate Mysteries: First, it is essential to assess the quantity of qi and blood followed by observing the arrival of qi. A light, smooth, and slow sensation beneath the needle indicates that qi hasn't yet arrived, while a heavy, unsmooth, and tight sensation signifies that qi has arrived. After the arrival of qi, the decision to retain the needle or remove it quickly should be based on the presence of cold or heat conditions. Prior to the arrival of qi, one must wait for its presence according to whether the condition is deficient or excessive. When qi arrives, it feels like the floating and sinking sensation of a fish taking the bait; if qi hasn't yet come, it resembles the emptiness experienced in a secluded hall. Acupuncture will take effect quickly if qi arrives promptly; however, if qi arrives slowly, the disease will be more difficult to cure.

The description of the practitioner's sensation during manipulation in *A Verse to Elucidate Mysteries* written by Dou Mou in the Yuan Dynasty has long been regarded as a classic account of Deqi. When Deqi is obtained, the practitioner may experience a heavy, unsmooth, and tight sensation or the feeling of a fish taking the bait of the needle. In the absence of Deqi, there will be a light, smooth, and slow sensation, similar to the emptiness one feels when staying in a large hall or quiet room.

Dou Mou believed that after Deqi is achieved, further needling manipulations should be determined based on the conditions of the disease. Additionally, the speed of the arrival of qi can be used to assess the prognosis.

KNOWLEDGE DATABASE: CULTURE

Lyric Poem and Verse (Gē Fù, 歌赋)

The lyric poem (Gē, 歌), also known as singable lyrics (Gē Xíng, 歌行) in Chinese and sometimes translated as ode or song, is an ancient form of poetry characterized by relatively free syllables and rhythms.

The verse (Fù, 赋) is another ancient Chinese literary style that emphasizes literary grace and rhythm. It possesses the beauty of both rhyme and prose.

Lyric poems and verses were used by ancient acupuncturists to summarize their experiences and educate students. A significant body of acupuncture literature in these two styles emerged after the Yuan Dynasty. Works such as *A Verse to Elucidate Mysteries*, *A Verse of Xi Hong* (see below) and *A Verse of Gold Needle* (see below), all of which are mentioned in this topic, appeared after the Yuan Dynasty and had a considerable influence during that time.

2.6 *The Complete Compendium of Acupuncture and Moxibustion*

Volume 1: A Verse of Xi Hong (*Juàn Yī · Xí Hóng Fù*, 卷一 · 席弘赋): When there's a sensation of numbness and heaviness, reducing techniques should be applied. If Deqi is achieved, it's not necessary to retain the needle.

Volume 5: A Verse of Gold Needle: An Abstract of Methods of Accelerating qi in Meridians from Zi Qi Feng Gu (*Juàn Wǔ · Zǐ Qí Fēng Gǔ Fēi Jīng Zǒu Qì Cuō Yào Jīn Zhēn Fù*, 卷五 · 梓岐风谷飞经走气撮要金针赋): When qi arrives quickly, acupuncture takes effect quickly; when qi arrives slowly, acupuncture takes effect slowly. A good prognosis or poor prognosis, as well as a high or low status, can all be discerned from the sensations felt beneath the needle. The low are strong, the high are fragile, the good are unsmooth, and the poor are deficient. If qi does not arrive after a prolonged period of waiting, death becomes inevitable.

A Verse of Xi Hong is a work from the Xi Hong School, which originated in the early southern Song Dynasty and flourished during the Ming Dynasty. This school emphasized the use of reinforcing and reducing techniques in its practices. The numbness and heaviness mentioned in the verse refer to the sensations experienced by the patient. The verse suggests that retaining the needle is not necessary once qi has arrived.

The Complete Compendium of Acupuncture and Moxibustion written by Xu Feng during the Ming Dynasty, includes *A Verse of Gold Needle*, authored by an individual using the alias Quan Shi. This article also posits that the speed of qi arrival is related to the therapeutic effect, and that the prognosis would be very poor if Deqi couldn't be achieved.

This article also suggests that the practitioner's hand sensation can be used to assess the patient's condition and prognosis. In individuals engaged in manual labour, the practitioner's sensation beneath the finger will be pronounced, whereas in those involved in mental labour, it will be weaker. Achieving Deqi is generally easier in patients with a good prognosis, while it tends to be more challenging in those with severe conditions.

2.7 *Introduction to Medicine*

> *Volume 1: Acupuncture and Moxibustion*: Confronting and following: ... The heavy, tight, and full sensations experienced by the practitioner indicate the arrival of qi. If the patient experiences aching, this suggests an excess condition, while soreness indicates a deficiency. On the other hand, light, floating, weak, and free sensations in the practitioner suggest that qi hasn't yet arrived. Induce qi by flicking, protruding, pressing, and touching. If qi still doesn't arrive after employing these techniques, and the sensation of inserting the needle into the body feels like inserting it into a soft tofu, the prognosis is very poor.

In *Introduction to Medicine* written by Li Chan during the Ming Dynasty, the assessment of the arrival of qi and its relationship with prognosis is similar to what is described in *A Verse to Elucidate Mysteries*. In addition, the book discusses the patient's sensations of aching and soreness. Aching indicates an excess syndrome, while soreness suggests a deficiency syndrome.

2.8 *The Great Compendium of Acupuncture and Moxibustion*

> *Volume 4: Reinforcing and Reducing of Mr. Gao in Siming* (*Juàn Sì · Sì Míng Fāo Shì Bǔ Xiè*, 卷四 · 四明高氏补泻): The needle is retained in the deeper layer for an extended period until there's no feeling of distention or qi movement. At that point, the needle is manipulated as before. If the qi arrives and the sensation of it wrapping around the needle doesn't disappear, it indicates an excess condition.... If the needle can be pushed without feeling any stagnation or distension, it indicates a qi deficiency...
>
> *Volume 4: Questions and Answers on Confronting-Following and Reinforcing -Reducing of Meridians and Collaterals* (*Juàn Sì · Jīng Luò Yíng Suí Bǔ Xiè Shè Wéi Wèn Dá,* 卷四 · 经络迎随补泻设为问答): For all needling depths, stop further thrusting when a startle sensation is felt around the needle. All reinforcing and reducing manipulations are intended to achieve Guqi.

The sensations of needling described in *The Great Compendium of Acupuncture and Moxibustion* include the absence of distension, the persistent feeling of qi wrapping around the needle, and the absence of stagnation. These sensations can be used to determine excess and deficiency. The sensations involve both the practitioner and the patient.

The Great Compendium of Acupuncture and Moxibustion also states that the depth of needling should be determined by the sensation of "a startle around the needle", and that reinforcing and reducing manipulations use Guqi as the standard. This perspective is consistent with that found in *The Inner Classic*. "A startle around the needle" refers to a sensation experienced by the practitioner during manipulation. Later, some scholars believe that this feeling is caused by the twitching of muscles.

2.9 *The Inner Analects of Acupuncture and Moxibustion* (*Zhēn Jiǔ Nèi Piān*, 针灸内篇)

> When inserting the needle into an acupoint, the process should be performed gradually and leisurely. During the treatment of a disease, the practitioner should cease manipulation when the patient experiences soreness, numbness, aching, or sensations akin to these feelings, to a degree that he can no longer endure, because this is the source of the disease... It's preferable if the patient feels soreness or numb-aching sensations, because this indicates a shallow disease that is easier to cure. If the patient doesn't feel anything during the needle insertion, the disease is signified as being deep-located and difficult to treat.

In the Qing Dynasty, an individual known by the alias Jiang Shang Wai Shi authored the book *The Inner Analects of Acupuncture and Moxibustion*. This book discusses the sensations experienced by the patient during acupuncture, such as soreness, numbness, and aching. Meanwhile, it stated that when the patient experienced soreness, numbness, aching or similar sensations to an intolerable degree, the needling should be stopped. This concept is akin to the idea of "cease the treatment upon the arrival of qi" found in *The Inner Classic*.

The book also linked the patient's sensations to the prognosis. The presence of soreness, numbness, and aching indicates a mild condition with a favorable prognosis; conversely, if these sensations are absent, it suggests that the disease is more severe and difficult to treat.

KNOWLEDGE DATABASE: LITERATURE

The Inner Analects of Acupuncture and Moxibustion (*Zhēn Jiǔ Nèi Piān*, 针灸内篇)

The Inner Analects of Acupuncture and Moxibustion is a book on acupuncture and moxibustion, written around 1821 during the Qing Dynasty. The author known by the literary name Jiang Shang Wai Shi (江上外史), is not known by his real name.

Jiang Shang Wai Shi was connected to the renowned Ling family of acupuncturists. The Ling family from the Shuanglin area has been recognized as a well-known acupuncture and moxibustion family for generations. In the Qing Dynasty, Ling Shengchen (凌声臣), a descendant of the Ling family, passed down the family's acupuncture techniques to his daughter's son, Xuan Peijiu, who then taught the methods to Jiang Shang Wai Shi.

2.10 *Acupuncture and Moxibustion Therapy in China* (*Zhōng Guó Zhēn Jiǔ Zhì Liáo Xué*, 中国针灸治疗学)

> *Volume 3: Manipulations of Acupuncture and Moxibustion* (*Dì Sān Biān · Zhēn Jiǔ Zhī Shī Yòng Fǎ*, 第三编 · 针灸之施用法): ... With this approach, the patient will experience only soreness, numbness, and a sensation of qi movement, without any pricking sensation from the needle.
>
> *Volume 3: Manipulations of Acupuncture and Moxibustion* (*Dì Sān Biān · Zhēn Jiǔ Zhī Shī Yòng Fǎ*, 第三编 · 针灸之施用法): ...Meanwhile, ask the patient if he can feel the onset of soreness and heaviness. If the patient only feels pain or neither soreness nor heaviness, the needle can be slightly thrust inwards or lifted outwards and then twisted. When the patient experiences soreness or heaviness and the practitioner feels a tight sensation around the needle, it indicates that the qi has arrived. At this point, reinforcing and reducing techniques can be applied.

In the 1930s, Cheng Dan'an wrote *Acupuncture and Moxibustion Therapy in China*, where he described the normal sensations that patients should experience after needling as "soreness, numbness, and qi movement". He stated that the feeling of "aching" wasn't considered a normal sign of the arrival of qi. During the manipulations, the practitioner should ask the patient if they feel "soreness and heaviness". If the patient does experience these sensations, it indicates that the qi has arrived, and reinforcing and reducing techniques can be applied.

KNOWLEDGE DATABASE: HISTORY

The Period of The Republic of China (中华民国时期)

The Republic of China period is often regarded as the first democratic republic in China, established after 1911. It lasted from 1912 to 1949 and served as a transitional period between the Qing Dynasty and modern China, known as the People's Republic of China.

KNOWLEDGE DATABASE: LITERATURE

***Acupuncture and Moxibustion Therapy in China* (*Zhōng Guó Zhēn Jiǔ Zhì Liáo Xué*, 中国针灸治疗学)**

Acupuncture and Moxibustion Therapy in China was first published in 1931 in the Republic of China period, and within less than 10 years, it went through 8 editions. The author Cheng Dan'an wrote this book with the aim of making the traditional theory of acupuncture scientific. In it, he introduced concepts from modern medicine, including anatomy, physiology, and pathology and began to establish a modern system of acupuncture and moxibustion.

3. Note

In contemporary acupuncture literature, the concept of "Deqi" or "arrival of qi" has evolved different from the pulse diagnosis discussed in *The Inner Classic*. Therefore, the notion that "the effect is achieved upon the arrival of qi" in *The Inner Classic* cannot be directly applied to modern clinical practice. The emergence of acupuncture is closely linked to pulse diagnosis, and in clinical practice, pulse diagnosis is often understood as the assessment of the Cunkou pulse. In addition, its specific application in acupuncture clinic can vary significantly. Acupuncture treatment must emphasize the use of palpation, inspection, and other methods to assess the flow of meridians. It is essential to pay attention to any abnormal reactions in the meridians, collaterals, and minute collaterals, as these observations provide the foundation for effective acupuncture.

Reflections

(1) What is the relationship between the arrival of Guqi, the arrival of qi and Deqi? How can practitioners achieve "the arrival of qi"? How can they determine when "the arrival of qi" has occurred?

(2) What is the difference between the connotations of "the arrival of qi" in *The Inner Classic* and "Deqi" in contemporary *Techniques of Acupuncture and Moxibustion*?

(3) Why did the concept of the "arrival of qi" in *The Inner Classic* evolve into the contemporary notion of "Deqi"? What are the advantages of each in clinical practice, and can they be used together?

Terms and Synonyms

(1) History, culture and people

Term	Chinese	Explanations
The Republic of China period	中华民国	The period from 1912 to 1949 in China
Lyric poem and verse	歌 赋	Ancient Chinese literary styles

(continued)

Term	Chinese	Explanations
Wang Huaiyin	王怀隐	One of the authors of *Formulas from Benevolent Sages Compiled during the Taiping Era*
Jiang Shang Wai Shi	江上外史	The alias of the author of *The Inner Analects of Acupuncture and Moxibustion*
Cheng Dan'an	承淡安	The author of *Acupuncture and Moxibustion Therapy in China*

(2) Acumox techniques

Term	Synonym	Chinese
Deqi	• Arrival of qi • Obtaining qi	得　气
	Needling sensation	针　感
Soreness, distension, heaviness and numbness		酸胀重麻
Transmitting and radiating feeling		放射、传导感
Sinking, tight or unsmooth feelings		沉涩紧

(3) Book names

Term	Synonym	Chinese
Formulas from Benevolent Sages Compiled during the Taiping Era	*Tai Ping Shen Hui Fang*	太平圣惠方
The Inner Analects of Acupuncture and Moxibustion	*Zhen Jiu Nei Pian*	针灸内篇
Acupuncture and Moxibustion Therapy in China	*Zhong Guo Zhen Jiu Zhi Liao Xue*	中国针灸治疗学
A Verse to Elucidate Mysteries	*Biao You Fu*	标幽赋
A Verse of Xi Hong	*Xi Hong Fu*	席弘赋
A Verse of Gold Needle (An Abstract of *Methods of Accelerating qi in Meridians from Zi Qi Feng Gu*)	*Jin Zhen Fu*	金针赋
	Zi Qi Feng Gu Fei Jing Zou Qi Cuo Yao Jin Zhen Fu	梓岐风谷飞经走气撮要金针赋

(4) Issues of *The Classic of Questioning*

Term	Pinyin & Chinese	Main Contents
The 70th Issue	七十难	Acupuncture techniques
The 78th Issue	七十八难	Acupuncture techniques

Topic 3

Moxibustion

1. General concepts of moxibustion

Moxibustion is a therapy that involves the use of inflammable materials, such as mugwort leaves or other heat-producing substances, to burn or warm acupoints or affect areas of the body.

Moxibustion is classified into two main types: moxibustion with moxa and moxibustion with other materials. Moxibustion with moxa includes direct moxibustion, such as scarring moxibustion, which uses moxa cones and various forms of insulated moxibustion. It also encompasses suspended moxibustion, which employs a normal moxa roll, and pressing moxibustion, which utilizes the Taiyi Miraculous Needle and the Thunder-Fire Needle. Additionally, warming needle moxibustion is also included. Moxibustion with other materials includes techniques using rush or mulberry twigs and certain types of natural moxibustion that involve stimulating medicinal materials.

2. The development of moxibustion

2.1 The Qin and Han dynasties

The main type of moxibustion during the Qin and Han dynasties was direct moxibustion.

2.1.1 Silk books and bamboo-slip books

The Classic of Moxibustion on Eleven Meridians on the Feet and Arms: (The foot Taiyang vessel)... Diseases presenting these symptoms should all be treated with moxibustion on the Taiyang vessel.

The Classic of Moxibustion on Eleven Meridians of Yin and Yang: For the Shaoyin vessel, moxibustion on it can improve appetite and promote flesh growth. When combined with loosened belts, hair hanging freely, walking with the aid of a strong stick, and wearing heavy shoes, the disease will be cured when moxibustion treatment is discontinued.

Formulas for Fifty-two Diseases (*Wǔ Shí Èr Bìng Fāng*, 五十二病方): The newt: ... Apply mustard to the center of the wound.

Formulas for Fifty-two Diseases: The wart: Cattail stems, when poorly or thickly matted, are fashioned into a fine rope. This rope can be ignited at one end and used for moxibustion directly on the wart. When the patient feels heat, the wart can be pulled out and removed.

Formulas for Fifty-two Diseases: (Hernia): Hemp ash wrapped in moxa can be used for moxibustion at the center of the hernia. This treatment will cause the hernia to ulcerate and eventually heal.

The Book of Vessels (*Mài Shū*, 脉书): If qi rises and does not descend, identify the affected vessel. Apply moxibustion to the vessel at the wrist or ankle. For severe cases, additional moxibustion should be applied to the area two *cun* above the wrist or ankle.

There're 11 vessels recorded in the *Classic of Moxibustion on Eleven Meridians on the Feet and Arms* and *The Classic of Moxibustion on Eleven Meridians of Yin and Yang*. The therapeutic approach for diseases of these vessels involves "moxibustion on the XX vessel". Similar information is recorded in other silk manuscripts. This is the earliest known medical text to document the therapy of moxibustion. The *Formulas for Fifty-two Diseases* and *Methods of the Vessel* [1], which were unearthed alongside the previous two texts, also mention moxibustion. However, these references are not on meridians, but to specific areas of the body, such as "the middle toe of the foot", etc.

At that time, moxibustion was typically performed by burning the skin with mild fire, and the materials used included hemp, mugwort, and cattail, etc. There was also a method involving the application of medicinal substances to specific areas of the body, which later came to be known as "cold moxibustion" or "natural moxibustion".

KNOWLEDGE DATABASE: LITERATURE

Formulas for Fifty-two Diseases (*Wǔ Shí Èr Bìng Fāng*, 五十二病方)

Formulas for Fifty-two Diseases refers to one of the silk books unearthed from the Mawangdui tombs of

1. The last excerpt above can be found in both *The Book of Vessels* from the Zhangjiashan tombs and *Methods of the Vessel* from the Mawangdui tombs. While the latter is incomplete, the former offers a different and more comprehensive version of the text. Therefore, the text from the Zhangjiashan tombs is used here.

the Han Dynasty. It's the earliest extant medical prescription book, containing a list of 52 diseases in its contents.

In addition to oral methods, the book also details various external treatment methods such as moxibustion, bian-stone therapy, hot compress, and fumigation.

2.1.2 *Huangdi's Inner Classic*

> *The Meridians* of *The Spiritual Pivot*: The sinking should be treated with moxibustion.
>
> *Employment of Ability* of *The Spiritual Pivot* (*Líng Shū · Guān Néng*, 灵枢 · 官能): When acupuncture can't be used to treat the condition, moxibustion should be applied.
>
> *Back-Shu Points* of *The Spiritual Pivot* (*Líng Shū · Bèi Shù*, 灵枢 · 背腧): Use reducing techniques if qi is excessive, and reinforcing techniques if qi is deficient. When using moxibustion to tonify, the flame shouldn't be blown out but allowed to burn itself out. When using moxibustion to reduce, the fire should be quickly blown out, and the moxa cone should be adjusted with the hand to ensure that the fire burns out quickly.
>
> *Discussion on Different Therapeutic Methods Suitable for Different Areas* of *Basic Questions* (*Sù Wèn · Yì Fǎ Fāng Yí Lùn*, 素问 · 异法方宜论): Cold in the zang organs can lead to fullness diseases, which should be treated with moxibustion. Therefore, moxibustion originates from the north.
>
> *Discussion on the Bone Holes* of *Basic Questions*: To treat cold-febrile diseases with moxibustion, begin by applying treatment to Dazhui at the nape of the neck, determining the number of cones based on the patient's age. Next, apply moxibustion to the coccyx, with the number of cones also determined by the patient's age.

In *The Inner Classic*, both acupuncture and moxibustion were utilized. According to the *Discussion on Different Therapeutic Methods Suitable for Different Areas* of *Basic Questions*, moxibustion originated from the north. The material used was moxa, and it's noted that moxibustion could be applied to diseases where acupuncture might not be suitable. In addition, the principles of reinforcing and reducing through moxibustion were illustrated. In *The Inner Classic*, the concept of "age-dependent *zhuang*", where the moxibustion dosage is determined based on age, was introduced. This was the first instance of "zhuang" being used as a measurement for moxibustion.

KNOWLEDGE DATABASE: LITERATURE

Employment of Ability of *The Spiritual Pivot* (*Líng Shū · Guān Néng*, 灵枢 · 官能): The 73rd chapter of the *Ling Shu*. It mainly explores the fundamentals of acupuncture, emphasizes the importance of early treatment and discusses the education of students based on their individual characteristics and abilities.

Back-Shu Points of *The Spiritual Pivot* (*Líng Shū · Bèi Shù*, 灵枢 · 背腧): The 51st chapter of the *Ling Shu*. It introduces the locations of back-Shu points and discusses the reinforcing and reducing techniques of moxibustion.

Discussion on Different Therapeutic Methods Suitable for Different Areas of *Basic Questions* (*Sù Wèn · Yì Fǎ Fāng Yí Lùn*, 素问 · 异法方宜论): The 12nd chapter of the *Su Wen*. It emphasizes that various therapeutic methods should be tailored to the specific needs of people from different regions.

2.2 The periods of the Jin, Sui, Tang, Song, Kin and Yuan dynasties

From the Jin to the Yuan Dynasties, moxibustion saw significant development. In addition to direct moxibustion, techniques such as stuff-insulated moxibustion, moxibustion with moxa-roll, and natural moxibustion were introduced, along with further elaborations on moxibustion dosage. Moxibustion was utilized both for treating and preventing diseases. During this period, the instruments used for moxibustion also began to take shape.

2.2.1 *The Systematic Classic of Acupuncture and Moxibustion*

Volume 3: ...Apply three *zhuang* of moxibustion.

Volume 3: To promote the suppuration, apply a hot compress using a sole warmed by moxibustion, and the sore will begin to suppurate within three days.

Volume 8: Apply moxibustion to the dog bite wounds, using three cones of moxibustion according to the method for treating dog bite injuries.

Acupoints listed in *Volume 3* of *The Systematic Classic of Acupuncture and Moxibustion* are derived from *The Therapeutic Importance of Acupuncture Points from the Bright Hall*. For each acupoint, both acupuncture and moxibustion techniques are described, with moxibustion typically involving 3 *zhuang* and at most 9 *zhuang*. At the end of volume 3, a method is proposed to promote the suppuration of moxibustion sores. In volume 8, the use of moxibustion cones for treating dog bites is discussed, specifying that the cones should be made from Chinese mugwort used for moxibustion.

2.2.2 *Emergency Formulas to Keep Up One's Sleeve* (*Zhǒu Hòu Bèi Jí Fāng*, 肘后备急方)

Preface: It requires specific needling techniques, but aside from those learning medical texts and understanding the principles of acupuncture theory, many people don't even know the locations of the ying qi and wei qi in the body. How can they effectively use needles to treat diseases? ... Additionally, when combined with moxibustion, only the locations are mentioned, without listing the names of the acupoints.

Volume 1: The 1st Collection of Formulas on Treating Sudden Stroke and Critical Collapse (*Juàn Yī · Jiù Cù Zhòng È Sǐ Fāng Dì Yī*, 卷一·救卒中恶死方第一): For sudden collapse with the eyes and mouth open, after applying moxibustion to both hands and feet...

Volume 2: The 12th Collection of Formulas on Treating Sudden Cholera and Various Emergencies (*Juàn Èr · Zhì Cù Huò Luàn Zhū Jí Fāng Dì Shí Èr*, 卷二·治卒霍乱诸急方第十二): Place salt into the navel and apply 14 *zhuang* of moxibustion.

Volume 2: The 13th Collection of Formulas on Treating Febrile Diseases, Epidemic Diseases, and Warm Diseases (*Juàn Èr · Zhì Shāng Hán Shí Qì Wēn Bìng Fāng Dì Shí Sān*, 卷二·治伤寒时气温病方第十三): Fumigate the patient by burning moxa in a tube and directing the smoke towards the anus.

Volume 3: The 19th Collection of Formulas on Treating Various Emergencies Due to Wind Stroke (*Juàn Sān · Zhì Zhōng Fēng Zhū Jí Fāng Dì Shí Jiǔ*, 卷三·治中风诸急方第十九): If there's fixed dragging pain and numbness, form a small round pill from moxa leaves and place it in a tile-pot with holes. Block all the holes except for one. Position the affected area under the open hole of the pot, burn the moxa to fumigate the area, and it should soon be relieved.

Volume 5: The 36th Collection of Formulas on Treating Carbuncles, Mammary Abscess, and Various Toxic Swellings (*Juàn Wǔ · Zhì Yōng Jū Dù Rǔ Zhū Dú Zhǒng Fāng Dì Sān Shí Liù*, 卷五·治痈疽妒乳诸毒肿方第三十六): Methods for reducing swelling with moxibustion: Place a piece of single-clove garlic, about one-*fen* thick, on the swollen area. The moxa cone should be roughly the size of a Chinese parasol tree seed. Apply more than one hundred *zhuang* of moxibustion on the garlic. If the swelling doesn't subside, continue applying more moxibustion; the more, the better. Ensure it is not too hot. Lift the garlic if you feel pain. Replace the garlic when it becomes burnt. It is not necessary for the moxibustion to cause damage to the skin or flesh.

Volume 3: The 16th Collection of Formulas on Treating Various Nue of Chills and Fever (*Juàn Sān · Zhì Hán Rè Zhū Nuè Fāng Dì Shí Liù*, 卷三·治寒热诸疟方第十六): Before the suppuration occurs, crush some big monkshood and sift it through a sieve. Mix the powdered monkshood with some bitter alcohol, and apply the mixture to the back.

Emergency Formulas to Keep Up One's Sleeve, written by Ge Hong during the Jin Dynasty, is a medical book designed for emergencies. Unlike other texts of the time, it does not cover acupuncture techniques; instead, it focuses on treating emergencies with moxibustion, which was a significant innovation.

In addition to direct moxibustion techniques mentioned in early texts such as *The Inner Classic*, this book introduced insulated moxibustion methods for the first time, including garlic-insulated moxibustion and salt-insulated moxibustion, among others. Notably, the book emphasizes that it's not necessary to damage the skin or flesh, which makes insulated moxibustion more acceptable.

Some types of moxibustion involve the use of instruments. In these methods, tubes or tile-pots were used as containers, into which the moxa was placed to perform the moxibustion.

In *Emergency Formulas to Keep Up One's Sleeve*, in addition to the moxibustion methods mentioned earlier, there're some records of external applications using a mixture of big monkshood and bitter alcohol. This represents a further development of cold moxibustion from the pre-Qin period. However, there's no specific term for cold moxibustion or natural moxibustion in the text.

KNOWLEDGE DATABASE: LITERATURE

Emergency Formulas to Keep Up One's Sleeve (Zhǒu Hòu Bèi Jí Fāng, 肘后备急方)

Emergency Formulas to Keep Up One's Sleeve is a medical prescription book written by Ge Hong (c. 281–c. 341) of the Eastern Jin Dynasty. The book was originally composed of three volumes, which were later expanded to eight volumes by scholars in subsequent generations. This book is an emergency treatment manual characterized by its simplicity, convenience, accuracy, and cost-effectiveness. While it includes treatments for both acupuncture and moxibustion, moxibustion is the predominant method because Ge Hong believed that it was impractical for untrained individuals to use needles.

Emergency Formulas to Keep Up One's Sleeve has gained prominence in recent years due to artemisinin, an antimalarial agent isolated from the herb known as sweet wormwood by Chinese scientists. According to one of its main contributors, the isolation procedure for artemisinin was inspired by the book's record of sweet wormwood's use in treating malaria.

KNOWLEDGE DATABASE: CULTURE

Keep up One's Sleeves (Zhou Hou, 肘后)

The literal translation of "keep up one's sleeves" is "behind the elbow", referring to the area above the elbow inside the sleeves of traditional Chinese clothing where a small pocket can be found for carrying items.

The name *Emergency Formulas to Keep Up One's Sleeve* indicates that Ge Hong intended for the book to be easily portable so that its formulas and methods could be applied promptly in emergencies. Today, the term "Zhou Hou (肘后)" is commonly used to refer to items that can be carried on, particularly medical books or prescriptions.

2.2.3 *Sketch Formulas* (*Xiǎo Pǐn Fāng*, 小品方) (Collected)

> *Volume 12: Key Points of Moxibustion* (*Juàn Shí Èr · Jiǔ Fǎ Yào Xué*, 卷十二 · 灸法要穴): Huang Di said: If the moxibustion cone doesn't reach 3 *fen* in width, it's essentially cheating. Explanation: This refers to the size of the moxibustion cone, and it's required that the base of the cone have a width of 3 *fen* to be considered appropriate... Now, in the regions east of the Changjiang River and south of the Five Ridges, where there is more earth dampness and less wind cold, the width of the moxibustion cones should be within 2 *fen*, at most 1.5 *fen* which is based on the shape of the human body. For infants, the size of the cones should be determined with extra caution.
>
> ... For Juque (CV14) and Jiuwei (CV15), although they're located on the chest and abdomen, the number of moxibustion cones used should not exceed 7 times 7. The size of each moxa cone should be small, approximately the size of the tip of a bamboo chopstick...

Sketch Formulas was written by Chen Yanzhi in the second half of the 5th century but was lost after the Song Dynasty. Based on incomplete copy recently discovered in Japan and other medical literature, some scholars compiled a version of it. This book discusses the moxa cone, a moxibustion material shaped like a column made from moxa wool.

KNOWLEDGE DATABASE: LITERATURE

Sketch Formulas (*Xiǎo Pǐn Fāng*, 小品方) (Collected)

Sketch Formulas is a collected version of a long-lost book that was compiled in the second half of the 5th century by the author Chen Yanzhi. According to the author, the medical knowledge in this book is classified as Xiao Pin, which can be understood as minor or sketchy. The author suggested that this book was suitable for those who wanted to be prepared for emergencies. However, for those who wished to pursue a career in medicine, other books should be consulted.

The book had a significant influence in history, and although it was lost, some of its contents are preserved in various surviving documents. In 1985, fragments of this book were discovered in Japan, including the contents, which enabled the reconstruction of the whole book.

2.2.4 *Collective Commentaries on the Classic of Materia Medica* (*Běn Cǎo Jīng Jí Zhù*, 本草经集注)

> *Volume 4: Herbaceous and Woody Plants of Middle Class* (*Juàn Sì · Cǎo Mù Zhōng Pǐn*, 卷四 · 草木中品): The leaf of mugwort has a bitter flavour, is mildly warm, and is nontoxic. It can be used to treat various ailments through moxibustion and can also be prepared as a decoction... Its alternate names are Bing Tai (ice base) or Yi Cao (medical grass). Growing in the field, it should be harvested on the third of March and dried in the sun... The leaves can be crushed and used in moxibustion to treat various ailments, and they can also help stop bleeding from injuries.

In the *Collective Commentaries on the Classic of Materia Medica*, written by Tao Hongjing, the flavour and properties of the Chinese mugwort leaf are recorded in detail. It notes that when used in moxibustion, it can treat various diseases. The detailed method is as follows: The leaves are first dried in the sun and then crushed for use in moxibustion. This describes the processing and application of moxa wool.

KNOWLEDGE DATABASE: LITERATURE

Collective Commentaries on the Classic of Materia Medica (*Běn Cǎo Jīng Jí Zhù*, 本草经集注)

The *Collective Commentaries on the Classic of Materia Medica* was compiled by Tao Hongjing (c. 456–536) between 492 and 500. This book is the earliest known commentary on *Shen Nong's Classic of Materia Medica* (*Shén Nóng Běn Cǎo Jīng*, 神农本草经), one of the fundamental texts of TCM, which introduces Chinese materia medica. The current version of the *Collective Commentaries on the Classic of Materia Medica* is a compiled edition because the original book was long lost. Its main contents have been preserved in various surviving manuscripts.

2.2.5 *Treatise on the Origins and Manifestations of Various Diseases* (*Zhū Bìng Yuán Hòu Lùn*, 诸病源候论)

> *Volume 45: Manifestations of Various Infantile Diseases* (*Juàn Sì Shí Wǔ · Yǎng Xiǎo Èr Hòu*, 卷四十五 · 养小儿候): Be aware that preventive acupuncture and moxibustion should not be applied to healthy newborns... In the region between the Yellow River and the Luo River, which

is typically cold, children are prone to convulsions. Consequently, there is a practice of applying preventive moxibustion to 3-day-old newborns to help prevent these issues. Additionally, moxibustion is sometimes applied to the cheek to prevent lockjaw.

During the Sui Dynasty, Cao Yuanfang documented preventive acupuncture and moxibustion, with particularly detailed accounts of preventive moxibustion for newborns to avert diseases. This represents one method of moxibustion used for preventive purposes.

KNOWLEDGE DATABASE: LITERATURE

Treatise on the Origins and Manifestations of Various Diseases (Zhū Bìng Yuán Hòu Lùn, 诸病源候论)

Treatise on the Origins and Manifestations of Various Diseases is the earliest extant book that explores the causes and symptoms of diseases. Written by Chao Yuanfang (fl. 605–616) and others in 610 during the Sui Dynasty, the book is divided into 67 sections and describes 1,720 syndromes and symptoms. However, it does not include any treatment prescriptions.

2.2.6 *Important Formulas worth a Thousand Gold Pieces for Emergency*

Volume 29: No. 6, Moxibustion Rules (*Juàn Èr Shí Jiǔ · Jiǔ Lì Dì Lìu*, 卷二十九 · 灸例第六): If the moxibustion cone doesn't reach 3 *fen* in width, it will have no therapeutic effect and may only cause pain. ... When performing moxibustion, the patient should be positioned straight, ensuring that the four limbs are evenly balanced. If the point is not correctly located during moxibustion, it won't be effective and may even damage normal tissue. If the point is found while the patient is sitting, moxibustion should also be performed with the patient in a sitting position; if the point is located while the patient is lying down, moxibustion should be done in the lying position; and if the point is located while the patient is standing, moxibustion should be carried out with the patient standing. If the guidelines are not followed, the acupoint may not be correctly located. ... For diseases caused by external factors, fewer moxibustion cones should be used; whereas for diseases originating internally, a great number of moxibustion cones should be applied.... For individuals who travel to the Wu or Shu regions to serve as officials, frequent moxibustion on two or three areas of the body is necessary, and the resulting wounds should remain unhealed for some time. This practice helps prevent local miasma, pestilence, warm Nue, and toxic qi from affecting people. This is why moxibustion is particularly popular in the Wu and Shu regions.

Volume 23: No. 1, Nine Fistulas (*Juàn Èr Shí Sān · Jiǔ Lòu Dì Yī*, 卷二十三·九漏第一): The moxibustion method for treating fistulas involves using 2 *ge* of ting li zi (Semen Lepidii) and 1 *sheng* of fermented soy beans. The two herbs are mixed together and finely ground into a very refined state. Then, shape the mixture into a large cake approximately 2 *fen* thick. Place one piece of the prepared mixture into the hole of the sore and form a moxa cone about the size of a little finger. Perform cake-insulated moxibustion, changing the cake after every three cones, for a total of three cakes and nine cones. Repeat the moxibustion treatment 3 days later.

In *Important Formulas Worth a Thousand Gold Pieces for Emergency*, Sun Simiao proposed several therapeutic routines for moxibustion. For example, the moxa cone should have a diameter of 3 *fen*, the posture should be straight during moxibustion, and the number of moxa cones should be adjusted based on the specific disease being treated.

This book also presents methods for disease prevention using moxibustion, a practice commonly referred to as preventive moxibustion. This approach has been further developed in later periods.

Besides, this book further elaborates on insulated moxibustion by introducing medicinal cake-insulated moxibustion. This involves using a cake made from semen Lepidii and fermented soy bean as insulation.

KNOWLEDGE DATABASE: CULTURE

Ge (合), Sheng (升)

Ge (合) and Sheng (升) are both units of volume. One sheng is equivalent to ten ge.

Other commonly used units of volume include dan (石) and dou (斗). One dan is equivalent to ten dou, and one dou is equivalent to ten sheng.

2.2.7 *Arcane Essentials from the Imperial Library*

Volume 39: Preface to the Bringh Hall: (The needle) can kill the living but cannot rescue the dead. I want to include this in the book, but I worry that it might pose a risk to life. Therefore, I won't copy the needle classics and will only record moxibustion.

Volume 30: 7 Formulas for Itching Due to Scabies (*Juàn Sān Shí · Jiè Fēng Yǎng Fāng Qī Shǒu*, 卷三十 · 疥风痒方七首): Prepare some moxa about the size of an egg. First, wrap some hair in a piece of cloth. Then, place the moxa, realgar powder, cinnabar powder, almond powder, and mercury, each the size of an almond, onto the paper. Ground the mercury in the palm with saliva and spread it on the paper to form a medicinal powder roll. Bake the roll until it is dry, and then burn it for fumigation.

Volume 39: Discussion on Moxibustion for Wind Cold Heat Due to Evil Invading Skin, Hair, Meridians, and Collaterals (*Juàn Sān Shí Jiǔ · Lùn Xié Rù Pí Máo Jīng Luò Fēng Lěng Rè Jiǔ Fǎ*, 卷三十九 · 论邪入皮毛经络风冷热灸法): ... The sun flint or fire pearl can be used to ignite a fire by reflecting sunlight.... If the sore doesn't suppurate, the disease can't be cured.

Wang Tao held a prejudice against needling techniques, so his book, *Arcane Essentials from the Imperial Library*, only collected the therapy of moxibustion. His views had a significant impact on subsequent practices of moxibustion. Following his work, there're a dozen moxibustion monographs, for example, *Moxibustion Techniques for Emergency* (*Bèi Jí Jiǔ Fǎ*, 备急灸法).

In *Arcane Essentials from the Imperial Library*, the method for treating scabies by burning a mixture of moxa and medicinal powders wrapped in paper is described. This technique involved a type of moxa stick that contained medicine. The Tai Yi Miraculous Needle and the Thunder-Fire Needle in later periods were similar to this one. This book also presented the method of sun flint moxibustion and the view that suppuration is necessary for treating moxibustion sores.

2.2.8 *Moxibustion Techniques for Gaohuangshu* (*Jiǔ Gāo Huāng Shù Xué Fǎ*, 灸膏肓俞穴法)

Postscript: Apply moxibustion to Gaohuangshu... After treatment, the disease gradually improved, and I eventually recovered.... Consequently, I examine medical classics to identify their similarities and differences. Based on other doctors' theories and my own experience, I divided my book into 10 chapters, ranging from point location by unit measurement to nourishing methods.

Zhuang Chuo's persistent illness was cured through moxibustion on Gaohuang (BL43). Consequently, he gathered related materials and wrote the book *Moxibustion Techniques for Gaohuangshu*. This book provides detailed records on the location of Gaohuang (BL43) and various moxibustion methods, along with post-moxibustion care techniques. It is recognized as the first book dedicated to single-point moxibustion.

KNOWLEDGE DATABASE: LITERATURE

***Moxibustion Techniques for Gaohuangshu* (*Jiǔ Gāo Huāng Shù Xué Fǎ*, 灸膏肓俞穴法)**

Moxibustion Techniques for Gaohuangshu was written by Zhuang Chuo (fl. 1127–1128) around 1128 during the Southern Song Dynasty. The book is quite unique as it focuses solely on one method—moxibustion techniques—applied just to one point—Gaohuang (BL43). This is attributed to the author's personal experience. Zhuang Chuo was not a doctor but an official. He suffered from a disease and tried various treatments, none of which were effective. Finally, he received 300 cones of direct moxibustion on Gaoguang (BL43) over the course of 7 days, leading to significant improvement. After receiving additional moxibustion treatments on Gaohuang (BL43), he was finally cured. Later, his relatives and friends also benefited greatly from this method. Consequently, Zhuang Chuo gathered information, including the location of Gaohuang (BL43) and the details of moxibustion techniques, and compiled this book.

2.2.9 *The Teachings of Bian Que* (*Biǎn Què Xīn Shū*, 扁鹊心书)

> *Volume 1: Advisable Treatment of Moxibustion in Serious Diseases* (*Juàn Shàng · Dà Bìng Yí Jiǔ*, 卷上・大病宜灸): Only high-fed people can't endure the pain. They can take "sleeping saint powder", which will cause them to lose consciousness and not feel the pain.

In *The Teachings of Bian Que*, Dou Cai mentioned that "sleeping saint powder" can be used as an adjuvant medicine to alleviate the pain caused by direct moxibustion.

KNOWLEDGE DATABASE: LITERATURE

***The Teachings of Bian Que* (*Biǎn Què Xīn Shū*, 扁鹊心书)**

The Teachings of Bian Que was written by Dou Cai in 1146 during the Southern Song Dynasty. This 3-volume comprehensive medical book includes treatments for various diseases and provides methods of moxibustion for both therapeutic and preventive purposes. This book proposes for the first time the use of "Sleeping Saint Powder", an anesthetic formula made from herbs, which can be taken before moxibustion to induce drowsiness and make individuals unaware of the pain associated with the procedure.

KNOWLEDGE DATABASE: CULTURE

Bian Que (扁鹊), Ling Ying (灵应), Shen Ying (神应)

Bian Que (扁鹊) was a famous ancient Chinese physician. During the Song Dynasty and subsequent periods, his name gained prominence. This was partly because, in the Song Dynasty, a doctor named Xu Xi cured an emperor with acupuncture and was subsequently rewarded. Xu Xi claimed that all his skills were derived from Master Bian Que, which led the emperor to grant Xu Xi's request to build a temple for Bian Que. Besides, the emperor also conferred the title of "Marquis Ling Ying (灵应侯)" upon Bian Que, with "Ling Ying" meaning "miraculous effect". In subsequent periods, the names of Bian Que and titles like Ling Ying (or similar "Shen Ying" (神应) became widely recognized in medical books, especially in texts concerning acupuncture.

2.2.10 *Classic of Nourishing Life with Acupuncture and Moxibustion*

> *Volume 3: Nue Spleen Coldness* (*Juàn Sān · Nuè Pí Hán*, 卷三 · 疟脾寒): People living in the countryside will crush han lian cao (herba Ecliptae) and place it about 1-fu the length of four fingers above the palm, between two tendons. Then they press it down with an ancient coin and secure it with a piece of used silk cloth. Small blisters will soon appear, and this method is known as natural moxibustion.

In the *Classic of Nourishing Life with Acupuncture and Moxibustion*, written by Wang Zhizhong during the Southern Song Dynasty, the practice of natural moxibustion using han lian cao was recorded. Following this, the use of natural moxibustion became increasingly widespread.

2.2.11 *Categorized Outline of the Causes and Manifestations of Cold Damage* (*Shāng Hán Biāo Běn Xīn FǎLèi Cuì*, 伤寒标本心法类萃)

> *Volume 2: Formulae* (*Juàn Xià · Fāng*, 卷下 · 方): The Taiyi Miraculous Needle includes the following ingredients: 4 *liang* each of qiang huo, duo huo, and huang lian (all in powder form), along with 2 *qian* each of she xiang and ru xiang. Moxa leaves, collected on March 3 or April 8, are dried in the sun and processed into moxa wool. Mix the moxa wool with the medicinal powder thoroughly, and then wrap the mixture in good-quality white paper, cut to the size of a chopstick. This can be used to treat wind-bi syndrome in the leg, waist, or arm. Using 7, 14, or 21 cones will yield quite effective results.

Liu Wansu recorded the method for making the Taiyi Miraculous Needle, which is a type of moxibustion using moxa sticks.

KNOWLEDGE DATABASE: LITERATURE

***Categorized Outline of the Causes and Manifestations of Cold Damage* (*Shāng Hán Biāo Běn Xīn Fǎ Lèi Cuì*, 伤寒标本心法类萃)**

Categorized Outline of the Causes and Manifestations of Cold Damage is a 2-volume work discussing cold damage (febrile diseases). The original edition attributes the authorship to Liu Wansu, but this book is often regarded as pseudonymous and may not be Liu's original creation.

Liu Wansu (c. 1110–1200) was one of the four famous doctors of the Jin and Yuan dynasties. He is well-known for his fire-heat theory, which posits that all six qi can transform into fire.

KNOWLEDGE DATABASE: HISTORY

The Jin Dynasty

The Jin Dynasty (金朝、金代) ruled from 1115 to 1234. To avoid confusion with the earlier Jìn dynasty (266–420), which shares the same pinyin without tone markings, this dynasty is sometimes written as Kin, Jinn, or Chin in English.

The Jin Dynasty preceded the Yuan Dynasty. In fact, the Jin Dynasty and the Southern Song Dynasty, which lasted from 1127 to 1279, coexisted for much of that period. This was because the Southern Song lost control of northern China to the Jin, leading to Song rule in the south and Jin rule in the north. Together, they governed China for over a century before being sequentially conquered by the Yuan Dynasty.

KNOWLEDGE DATABASE: CULTURE

Liang (两), Qian (钱)

Liang (两) and Qian (钱) are both units of weight. One liang equals 10 qian. Fen, which is a unit of length mentioned before, can also be a unit of weight. 1 qian equals 10 fen.

Another commonly used unit of weight is the jin (斤). One jin equals 10 liang.

2.2.12 *Moxibustion for Emergency* (*Bèi Jí Jiǔ Fǎ*, 备急灸法)

Moxibustion on A Bamboo-horse (*Qí Zhú Mǎ Jiǔ Fǎ*, 骑竹马灸法): The diameter of the moxa cone should be three *fen*. The cone is made from moxa rolled into a long shaft and wrapped in paper. It should be used only when it's very tight packed....The moxa is tightly rolled with paper into a shaft, which can then be cut into cones.

The method of making moxa cones is not commonly found in early literature. It was not until the Song Dynasty's *Moxibustion for Emergency* that the process was documented. The method involved first creating moxa sticks, which could then be cut into sections for further use.

KNOWLEDGE DATABASE: LITERATURE

***Moxibustion for Emergency* (*Bèi Jí Jiǔ Fǎ*, 备急灸法)**

Moxibustion for Emergency is a one-volume book written by Wenren Qinian in 1226 during the Southern Song Dynasty. It covers moxibustion treatments for around 20 emergent conditions. In 1245, the book was republished along with *Moxibustion on A Bamboo-Horse* (*Qí Zhú Mǎ Jiǔ Fǎ*, 骑竹马灸法) and *Zhuge's Experiential Prescriptions for Emergency* (*Zhú Gé Jīng Yàn Bèi Jí Yào Fāng*, 竹阁经验备急药方), but it continued to be referred to as *Moxibustion for Emergency*.

2.3 The period of Ming and Qing dynasties

During the Ming and Qing dynasties, moxibustion was further refined and improved. Techniques such as warming-needle moxibustion and moxibustion using instrument were enhanced and perfected.

2.3.1 *Mirror of Ancient and Modern Medical Works* (*Gǔ Jīn Yī Jiàn*, 古今医鉴)

Volume 13: Lumps (*Juàn Shí Sān · Pǐ Jí*, 卷十三 · 癖疾): The method for treating lumps with tendon-picking and moxibustion is as follows: ... Wipe the area with a piece of medicinally prepared paper to ensure that the skin and flesh are numb, then apply one cone of moxibustion... Method for preparing the paper: Grind a hornet's nest from a pepper tree into powder. Rub the paper repeatedly with beeswax mixed with the powder and sesame oil. Then, use this paper to rub the skin of the affected area, which will become numb and insensitive to pain.

Volume 13: Lumps: ...Each point is treated with three coins, with the moxa cone placed in the hole created by stacking the coins. Seven cones are used for each point.

In the Ming Dynasty, Gong Xin recorded local anesthesia in his *Mirror of Ancient and Modern Medical Works*, which could help alleviate pain caused by acupuncture and moxibustion. The book also describes a technique using coins as the moxibustion instrument.

KNOWLEDGE DATABASE: LITERATURE

***Mirror of Ancient and Modern Medical Works* (*Gŭ Jīn Yī Jiàn*, 古今医鉴)**

Mirror of Ancient and Modern Medical Works is a comprehensive medical text from the Ming Dynasty. Compiled by Gong Xin, it was first published as an 8-volume book in 1576. In 1589, it was continued and republished by Gong Xin's son, Gong Tingxian (1522–1619). The work was further edited and expanded to 16 volumes by Wang Kentang (c. 1552–1638), a Ming Dynasty physician.

2.3.2 *A Collection of Gems in Acupuncture and Moxibustion*

Volume 3: Warming Needle (*Juàn Sān · Wēn Zhēn*, 卷三 · 温针): Wang Jiezhai mentioned that recently, someone has been using a technique known as warming needle, which originates from the Chu people. The method is as follows: Insert the needle into the acupoint, cover the needle with a round cake made from fragrant bai zhi (Radix Angelicae dahuricae), and then warm the cake with moxa fumigation.

In *A Collection of Gems in Acupuncture and Moxibustion*, there's a record of a method similar to contemporary warming needle therapy. However, the author noted that in an ancient treatment routine, "In ancient times, moxibustion wouldn't be applied if acupuncture was used, and vice versa. The combination of acupuncture and moxibustion has never been seen". This method was considered suitable only for "poor people with low social status living in the mountains or remote areas, who suffered from diseases caused by wind-cold attacking the meridians and collaterals". According to the book, this method may occasionally be effective, but it's primarily used to promote qi circulation through the warming needle therapy, and "wouldn't be of any help to the disease itself".

2.3.3 *Introduction to Medicine*

Volume 1: Acupuncture and Moxibustion: Point Methods for Miscellaneous Diseases: ...For cold wind and damp bi syndrome, the point Huantiao (GB30) can be used, and in Yanglingquan (GB34) and Zusanli (ST36), needle tails can be burnt. For bi syndrome without numbness or itching, apply 3—5 moxa cones, each the size of a grain of rice, to the tail of the needle. Stop the treatment when the patient begins to feel pain.

In the note for "*Point Methods for Miscellaneous Diseases*" in *Introduction to Medicine*, Li Chan proposed that "in Yanglingquan (GB34) and Zusanli (ST36), the needle tails can be burnt", and added that "apply 3–5 moxa cones, each the size of a grain of rice, to the tail of the needle. Stop the treatment when the patient begins to feel pain". This method should be the same as the modern warming needle moxibustion.

2.3.4 *The Grand Compendium of Materia Medica* (*Běn Cǎo Gāng Mù*, 本草纲目)

> *The Section of Fire: Miraculous Needle Fire* (*Huǒ Bù · Shén Zhēn Huǒ*, 火部 · 神针火): To create the Miraculous Needle Fire on May 5, peach tree twigs growing toward the east are sharpened into wooden needles about the size of an egg and 5 or 6 *cun* in length, then dried. During application, the affected area is covered with 3–5 layers of tissue paper. Dip the needle into sesame oil, then ignite it and blow it out. Apply the needle while it's still hot. There's also another type of Thunder-Fire Miraculous Needle: mix 1 *liang* of processed moxa powder from the Qi area with 1 *qian* each of ru xiang (Olibanum), mo yao (Myrrha), chuan shan jia (Squama Manis), liu huang (Sulfur), xiong huang (Realgar), cao wu tou (Radix Aconiti kusnezoffii), chuan wu tou (Radix Aconiti), tao shu pi (peach bark) and 5 *fen* of she xiang (Moschus). Grind all ingredients into a powder and mix with the moxa. Cut thick paper into strips, spread the medicated moxa inside, and roll the paper tightly into a shape about the size of a finger and 3–4 *cun* in length. Place them into a bottle and bury the bottle underground for 7 days, then retrieve it. For application, ignite the needle using a lamp and then blow out the flame. Cover the affected area with 10 layers of paper, and apply the needle while it's still hot.
>
> *The Section of Fire: Fire of Lamp* (*Huǒ Bù · Dēng Huǒ*, 火部 · 灯火): ...Dip the rush in and out of sesame oil, then ignite it and apply it. This method is effective.

In *The Grand Compendium of Materia Medica*, Li Shizhen recorded the use of moxibustion with peach twigs as the material, as well as the Thunder-Fire Needle and Lamp fire moxibustion.

KNOWLEDGE DATABASE: LITERATURE

The Grand Compendium of Materia Medica **(*Běn Cǎo Gāng Mù*, 本草纲目)**

The Grand Compendium of Materia Medica was compiled by Li Shizhen and its first draft was completed in 1578 during the Ming Dynasty. Printed in 1596, the book catalogs the materia medica of traditional Chinese medicine known at that time, including plants, animals, and minerals believed to have medicinal properties.

2.3.5 *Comprehensive Medicine According to Master Zhang* (*Zhāng Shì Yī Tōng*, 张氏医通)

Volume 4: Panting (*Juàn Sì · Chuǎn*, 卷四 · 喘): For cold wheezing, moxibustion can be applied to Feishu (BL13), Gaohuang (BL43), and Tiantu (CV22). While some individuals may respond positively to this treatment, others may not.. During the three fu-periods of summer, applying bai jie zi (Semen sinapis) is generally effective. The formula is as follows: 1 *liang* of clean bai jie zi powder, 1 *liang* of yan hu suo (Rhizoma Corydalis), and 0.5 *liang* each of gan sui (Radix Euphorbiae kansui) and xi xin (Radix et Rhizoma asari). All of the above ingredients are mixed and ground into a fine powder. Add 0.5 *qian* of musk, then crush them until it is uniform. Mix the powder with ginger juice and apply it to Feishu (BL13), Gaohuang (BL43), Bailao (EX-HN15), and other relevant points. After application, don't remove it when numbness and pain occur. Instead, leave it on until you have burned about three sticks of incense. Reapply the treatment after 10 days. Repeat this process three times, and it can help eliminate the root of the diseases.

In the early Qing Dynasty, *Comprehensive Medicine According to Master Zhang*, written by Zhang Lu, recorded a method for treating cold wheezing using medicinal applications made from bai jie zi and other herbs, applied to Feishu (BL13) and Gaohuang (GB43) during the three fu-periods of summer. This method is the prototype of the modern three fu-period application. The term Fu (伏) or three fu (三伏) refers to the hottest days of summer.

KNOWLEDGE DATABASE: LITERATURE

Comprehensive Medicine According to Master Zhang (_Zhāng Shì Yī Tōng_, 张氏医通)

Comprehensive Medicine According to Master Zhang was written by Zhang Lu (1617–1699) in 1695 during the Qing Dynasty. It's a 16-volume comprehensive medical text.

2.3.6 *Secret Transmissions of Moxibustion* (*Jiǔ Fǎ Mì Chuán*, 灸法秘传)

Picture of Moxibustion Cup (*Jiǔ Zhǎn Tú*, 灸盏图): Currently, ginger-insulated moxibustion with a silver cup is considered safe. Those who wish to use this method should follow this example: The surrounding silver pieces should be slightly thicker, while the base should be thin and perforated with several holes. The bottom of the cup should have four feet, each about one *fen* high. Place the foot of the cup into the ginger slice, and also created several holes in the ginger that align with the cup's holes, allowing the medicinal qi to penetrate into the meridians, collaterals, and zang-fu organs.

Secret Transmissions of Moxibustion, a book from the Qing Dynasty, describes the moxibustion cup used in moxibustion therapy. The moxibustion box developed later was based on this design.

KNOWLEDGE DATABASE: LITERATURE

***Secret Transmissions of Moxibustion* (*Jiǔ Fǎ Mì Chuán*, 灸法秘传)**

Secret Transmissions of Moxibustion was published in 1883 during the Qing Dynasty. The book, handed down from Jin Ye-tian and compiled by Lei Shaoyi (c. 1833–1888), consists of one-volume and primarily focuses on information related to moxibustion.

3. Note

Early moxibustion methods primarily used various moxibustion materials to treat diseases through the warming effect after burning. Over time, advancements in medical knowledge expanded the range of available moxibustion materials, and the indications for moxibustion also grew. In practice, due to the limited science and technology of the time, the understanding of drug toxicity was still insufficient. Therefore, the composition or production process of some moxibustion materials may have included toxic substances, such as mercury. Consequently, these moxibustion materials should not be used blindly in clinical settings.

Reflections

What are the similarities and differences between the functions and indications of natural moxibustion and moxibustion using moxa?

Terms and Synonyms

(1) History, culture and people

Term	Chinese	Explanations
The Jin Dynasty	金 朝	The ruling dynasty from 1115 to 1234
Sheng	升	A unit of volume: 1 sheng equals 10 ge

(continued)

Term	Chinese	Explanations
Ge	合	A unit of volume
Liang	两	A unit of weight: 1 liang equals 10 qian
Qian	钱	A unit of weight
Keep up One's Sleeves	肘后	Originally referring to an area inside the sleeves behind the elbow, it later came to denote something that can be carried, especially medical books or prescriptions
Zhou Hou		
Behind the elbow		
Bian Que	扁鹊	A legendary doctor known for his miraculous therapeutic effects, often referenced in book titles after the Song Dynasty, particularly those related to acupuncture
Ling Ying	灵应	
Shen Ying	神应	
Ge Hong	葛洪	The author of *Emergency Formulas to Keep Up One's Sleeve*
Chen Yanzhi	陈延之	The author of *Sketch Formulas*
Tao Hongjing	陶弘景	The author of *Collective Commentaries on the Classic of Materia Medica*
Chao Yuanfang	巢元方	The author of *Treatise on the Origins and Manifestations of Various Diseases*
Zhuang Chuo	庄绰	The author of *Moxibustion Techniques for Gaohuangshu*
Dou Cai	窦材	The author of *The Teachings of Bian Que*
Liu Wansu	刘完素	The author of *Categorized Outline of the Causes and Manifestations of Cold Damage*
Wenren Qinian	闻人耆年	The author of *Moxibustion for Emergency*
Gong Xin	龚信	The author of *Mirror of Ancient and Modern Medical Works*
Zhang Lu	张璐	The author of *Comprehensive Medicine According to Master Zhang*
Lei Shaoyi	雷少逸	The author of *Secret Transmissions of Moxibustion*

(2) Acumox techniques

Term	Synonym	Chinese
Moxa wool	Moxa floss	艾绒
Moxa cone		艾炷

(continued)

Term	Synonym	Chinese
Moxa stick		艾 条
Direct moxibustion		直接灸
Insulated moxibustion	• Isolated moxibustion • Cushioned moxibustion	隔物灸
Lamp fire moxibustion	• Moxibustion with rush • Juncibustion	灯火灸
Warming needle moxibustion	Warm needling	温针灸
Natural moxibustion	Vesiculation moxibustion	• 天 灸 • 发泡灸
Taiyi Miraculous Needle	Taiyi moxa stick moxibustion	太乙神针
Thunder-Fire Needle	Thunder-Fire wonder moxibustion	雷火神针

(3) Acumox therapeutics

Term	Synonym	Chinese
Preventive moxibustion	Early moxibustion	逆 灸 预防保健灸

(4) Book names

Term	Synonym	Chinese
Formulas for Fifty-two Diseases	*Wu Shi Er Bing Fang*	五十二病方
Emergency Formulas to Keep Up One's Sleeve	*Zhou Hou Bei Ji Fang*	肘后备急方
Sketch Formulas	*Xiao Pin Fang*	小品方
Collective Commentaries on the Classic of Materia Medica	*Ben Cao Jing Ji Zhu*	本草经集注
Treatise on the Origins and Manifestations of Various Diseases	*Zhu Bing Yuan Hou Lun*	诸病源候论
Moxibustion Techniques for Gaohuangshu	*Jiu Gao Huang Shu Xue Fa*	灸膏肓俞穴法
The Teachings of Bian Que	*Bian Que Xin Shu*	扁鹊心书

(continued)

Term	Synonym	Chinese
Categorized Outline of the Causes and Manifestations of Cold Damage	*Shang Han Biao Ben Xin Fa Lei Cui*	伤寒标本心法类萃
Moxibustion for Emergency	*Bei Ji Jiu Fa*	备急灸法
Mirror of Ancient and Modern Medical Works	*Gu Jin Yi Jian*	古今医鉴
The Grand Compendium of Materia Medica	*Ben Cao Gang Mu*	本草纲目
Comprehensive Medicine According to Master Zhang	*Zhang Shi Yi Tong*	张氏医通
Secret Transmissions of Moxibustion	*Jiu Fa Mi Chuan*	灸法秘传

(5) Chapters of *The Inner Classic*

The Spiritual Pivot

Term	Synonym	Chinese
Back-Shu Points	*Bei Shu*	背 腧
Employment of Ability	*Guan Neng*	官 能

Basic Questions

Term	Synonym	Chinese
Discussion on Different Therapeutic Methods Suitable for Different Areas	*Yi Fa Fang Yi Lun*	异法方宜论

Chapter 3
Acumox Therapeutics

Guidance

Understand the various perspectives of doctors from past dynasties on prohibiting moxibustion for the heat syndrome and the use of preventive moxibustion.

Master the evolution of the concepts behind acupuncture therapeutic principles and the relationship between pulse diagnosis and acumox.

Topic 1

The Heat Syndrome and Moxibustion

1. General introduction

Moxibustion has a wide range of indications, but due to its characteristics, it's generally believed to be most effective for treating deficient, cold, or yin syndromes. Specifically, it is often used for chronic or prolonged diseases and conditions associated with insufficient yang qi.

The heat syndrome, in traditional Chinese medicine, refers to patterns characterized by a hot nature according to the eight-principle syndrome differentiation. This includes patterns with a hot nature manifested in various conditions such as externally contracted febrile diseases, febrile diseases due to internal injury, and external conditions like carbuncles, sores, and ulcers. Historically, there've been differing opinions on whether moxibustion can be used to treat heat syndromes. Some practitioners believe that moxibustion is contraindicated in cases of the heat syndrome, while others argue that the heat syndrome can be effectively treated with moxibustion. In recent years, many textbooks have classified the heat syndromes as either a contraindication or a condition that requires caution when applying moxibustion.

2. The development of moxibustion application in treating the heat syndrome

2.1 Silk books and bamboo-slip books

> *The Classic of Moxibustion on Eleven Vessels on the Feet and Arms*: (The foot Yangming vessel) and its related diseases...including hot sweating. Diseases with these manifestations should all be treated with moxibustion on the Yangming vessel.

> *The Book of Vessels*: (Carbuncles and swelling) with pus shouldn't be treated with moxibustion.

Moxibustion is used to treat various diseases in both of the silk texts, *The Classic of Moxibustion on Eleven Vessels on the Feet and Arms* and *The Classic of Moxibustion on Eleven Vessels of Yin and Yang*, which were unearthed from Mawangdui. In *The Classic of Moxibustion on Eleven Vessels on the Feet and Arms*, it's mentioned that "hot sweating" can be treated with moxibustion. However, the bamboo-slip book *The Book of Vessels*, unearthed from Zhangjiashan, specifies that carbuncles or swelling with pus are not suitable for moxibustion.

2.2 *The Inner Classic*

> *Ending and Beginning* of *The Spiritual Pivot*: In patients with insufficient qi, both Maikou and Renying are weak and don't correspond to their expected sizes. In these cases, both yin and yang are insufficient...can be treated with herbs of sweet flavour... Such cases should not be treated with moxibustion... When the pulses at both Renying and Maikou are more than three times stronger than usual, this condition is referred to as an overflow of both yin and yang. This occurs due to a failure in communication within the body, leading to the blockage of blood vessels. Consequently, qi cannot flow properly and ends up overflowing internally, which in turn impairs the five zang organs. Treating this condition with moxibustion can lead to additional complications.
>
> *The Meridians* of *The Spiritual Pivot*: The sinking should be treated with moxibustion.
>
> *Back-Shu Points* of *The Spiritual Pivot*: When using moxibustion to tonify, the flame shouldn't be blown out but allowed to burn itself out. When using moxibustion to reduce, the fire should be quickly blown out, and the moxa cone should be adjusted with the hand to ensure that the fire burns out quickly.
>
> *Employment of Ability* of *The Spiritual Pivot*: When acupuncture can't be used to treat the condition, moxibustion should be applied... In cases of deficiency in both yin and yang, moxibustion can be effectively utilized.
>
> *Carbuncles and Abscesses* of *The Spiritual Pivot* (*Líng Shū · Yōng Jū*, 灵枢 · 痈疽): Carbuncles that occur on the shoulder and upper limbs are known as superficial carbuncles. They appear red and black and should be treated promptly. It may include sweating throughout the body but won't impact the five zang organs. Moxibustion should be applied promptly four to five days after the

onset of the carbuncle.

Discussion on the Bone Holes of *Basic Questions*: To treat cold-febrile diseases with moxibustion, begin by applying treatment to Dazhui at the nape of the neck, determining the number of cones based on the patient's age. Next, apply moxibustion to the coccyx, with the number of cones also determined by the patient's age.

In *The Inner Classic*, it's proposed that moxibustion is indicated for conditions such as sinking, deficiency of both yin and yang, and diseases for which acupuncture is not suitable. In addition, it notes that moxibustion is not suitable for situations involving insufficiency or overflow of both yin and yang. For diseases such as carbuncles and cold-fever, which can be differentiated as the heat syndrome, there're also corresponding moxibustion therapies detailed in *The Spiritual Pivot* and *Basic Questions*. The reinforcing and reducing methods of moxibustion described in *The Spiritual Pivot* are the manipulation principles of modern reinforcing and reducing techniques of moxibustion.

According to the texts in *The Inner Classic*, there're records of both febrile diseases treated with moxibustion and cases when moxibustion is contraindicated for febrile diseases. This reflects the medical practice of that time, indicating that while moxibustion could be used for febrile diseases, improper use might lead to deterioration.

KNOWLEDGE DATABASE: LITERATURE

Carbuncles and Abscesses of *The Spiritual Pivot* (*Líng Shū · Yōng Jū*, 灵枢 · 痈疽): The 81st chapter of the *Ling Shu*. It mainly introduces the names, symptoms, treatment and prognosis of carbuncles and abscesses.

2.3 *Treatise on Cold Damage and Miscellaneous Diseases* (*Shāng Hán Zá Bìng Lùn*, 伤寒杂病论)

Volume 3: Part 2, Differentiation of the Pulse, Syndrome and Treatment of the Taiyang Diseases (*Juàn Sān · Biàn Tài Yáng Bìng Mài Zhèng Bìng Zhì Zhōng*, 卷三 · 辨太阳病脉证并治中): For floating pulse and severe fever, where moxibustion shouldn't be applied but is still used, this constitutes an excessive condition. If an excessive condition is treated as a deficiency, it will be aggravated by the heat, likely leading to symptoms such as a dry throat and vomiting of blood. Be cautious that a weak and rapid pulse should not be treated with moxibustion. Otherwise, the condition could worsen due to the fire exacerbating the evil, leading to increased vexation and reversal. This could aggravate both deficiency and excess, causing the blood to disperse within the vessels. Although the fire may be weak, it can still penetrate the interior aggressively, potentially damaging bones and tendons and hindering blood recovery. A floating pulse should be treated with the sweating therapy; if treated with moxibustion, the evil can't be expelled; instead, it will be intensified by the fire. This can lead to symptoms such as heaviness and numbness below the waist, a condition known as malpractice of fire therapy.

Treatise on Cold Damage provides detailed accounts of the malpractice and adverse outcomes resulting from the misuse of fire, including fire fumigation, burned needles, warmed needles, or hot compresses in the treatment of febrile diseases caused by cold injury. The contraindications for moxibustion primarily include the exterior heat syndrome, characterized by a "floating pulse and severe fever"; the deficient heat syndrome, indicated by a "weak and rapid pulse"; and the exterior syndrome, marked by a "floating pulse".

Due to the significant influence of the *Treatise on Cold Damage*, later practitioners often didn't thoroughly study these records. As a result, the guideline that "moxibustion is contraindicated in the treatment of heat syndrome" gradually took shape.

KNOWLEDGE DATABASE: LITERATURE

***Treatise on Cold Damage and Miscellaneous Diseases* (*Shāng Hán Zá Bìng Lùn*, 伤寒杂病论)**

***Treatise on Cold Damage* (*Shāng Hán Lùn*, 伤寒论)**

***Essentials from the Golden Cabinet* (*Jīn Guì Yào Lüè*, 金匮要略)**

Treatise on Cold Damage and Miscellaneous Diseases is a classical work of TCM, written by Zhang Zhongjing (c. 150–219) of the Eastern Han Dynasty. The original text was lost, but later generations compiled it into two key works: the 10-volume *Treatise on Cold Damage* and the 3-volume *Essentials from the Golden Cabinet*. The most important contribution of this work is its introduction of diagnostic and treatment principles based on symptom differentiation.

2.4 Emergency Formulas to Keep Up One's Sleeve

Volume 5: The 36th Collection of Formulas on Treating Carbuncles, Mammary Abscess and

Various Toxic Swellings (*Juàn Wǔ · Zhì Tōng Jū Dù Rǔ Zhū Dú Zhǒng Fāng Dì Sān Shí Liù*, 卷五·治痈疽妒乳诸毒肿方第三十六): To treat breast sores and various types of carbuncles on the back and breasts, apply one hundred moxa cones to the affected area... For a swollen area that is hard and deeply rooted, known as a stony carbuncle, treat it with one hundred moxa cones in the affected area.

Emergency Formulas to Keep Up One's Sleeve, written by Ge Hong, details treatments for various urgent conditions, including methods for managing heat syndromes in external diseases such as carbuncles on the back, recommending the application of over 100 moxa cones.

2.5 *Formulas worth a Thousand Gold Pieces*

Volume 19: No. 5, Bone Exhaustion of *Important Formulas Worth a Thousand Gold Pieces for Emergency* (*Bèi Jí Qiān Jīn Yào Fāng · Juàn Shí Jiǔ · Gǔ Jí Dì Wǔ*, 备急千金要方·卷十九·骨极第五): For motor impairment of the waist and back, tendon spasms and contractions, and deficient heat with blockage, apply moxibustion to the twenty-first vertebra, which is located 1.5 *cun* lateral to the midline. The number of moxa cones should be determined based on the patient's age.

Volume 28: No. 5, Carbuncles of *Supplement to "Important Formulas Worth a Thousand Gold Pieces"* (*Qiān Jīn Yì Fāng · Juàn Èr Shí Bā · Yōng Jū Dì Wǔ*, 千金翼方·卷二十八·痈疽第五): For all sudden illnesses, such as swollen waist, bone-attached carbuncles, wind carbuncles, swellings, boils, and moving toxic and hot swellings, apply moxibustion immediately upon noticing any abnormal sensations. This can lead to prompt relief and potential cure. If swelling has already formed, it's not necessary to apply moxibustion directly to the affected area. Instead, apply 5 moxa cones to the area on the first crease above the palm, between the two tendons. This treatment will lead to immediate relief. Apply moxibustion on the right side if the left side is affected, and on the left side if the right side is affected. For issues in the chest or gastric area, apply moxibustion to both hands. This approach can effectively address and cure all swellings.

Formulas Worth a Thousand Gold Pieces summarizes the experiences of early periods and indicates that moxibustion can be used to treat both deficient heat and excessive heat.

2.6 The Teachings of Bian Que

Volume 1: Moxibustion Methods from Huangdi (*Juàn Shàng · Huáng Dì Jiŭ Fǎ*, 卷上·黄帝灸法): For persistent fever, which may gradually develop into consumptive diseases in women after childbirth, apply 300 cones of moxibustion to the area below the navel immediately.

Dou Cai used moxibustion to treat persistent fever after childbirth to prevent the onset of consumptive diseases.

2.7 Classic of Nourishing Life with Acupuncture and Moxibustion

Volume 3: Consumption (*Juàn Sān · Láo Zhài*, 卷三·痨瘵): For consumptive diseases characterized by a feverish feeling in the palms and soles and often accompanied by night sweats, moxibustion is recommended... Apply moxibustion with a number of moxa cones equal to the patient's age plus one. This method has frequently shown effective results.

In the *Classic of Nourishing Life with Acupuncture and Moxibustion*, Wang Zhizhong recorded moxibustion methods for various deficient heat issues, such as hectic fever due to yin deficiency and consumptive diseases.

2.8 Collection of Writings on the Mechanism of Disease, Suitability of Qi, and the Safeguarding of Life as Discussed in the "Basic Questions" (Sù Wèn Bìng Jī Qì Yí Bǎo Mìng Jí, 素问病机气宜保命集)

Volume 3: No. 26, Discussion on Sores and Ulcers (*Juàn Xià · Chuāng Yáng Lùn Dì Èr Shí Liù*, 卷下·疮疡论第二十六): Sores and ulcers are categorized as conditions related to fire...For sores and ulcers that are slightly swollen, generally hard, without changes in skin color or visible vessels, and have a deep pulse but no pain, moxibustion should be applied externally until the condition is resolved and the evils are expelled. Conditions with pus should not be treated with moxibustion but can be addressed with needling. Superficial conditions should also not be treated with moxibustion. According to *The Classic*, sinking conditions can be treated with moxibustion.

For conditions with a feeble feeling of numbness and hardness but without pain, moxibustion should be applied immediately, as this indicates deeply intruding evils. However, be cautious not to use moxibustion for superficial sores and ulcers.

Volume 3: No. 32, Summary of Medication (Juàn Xià · Yào Luè Dì Sān Shí Èr, 卷下 · 药略第三十二): Bone fever, which is difficult to cure, and dry front teeth can be treated with moxibustion at Dazhui (GV14), where the bones converge.

Liu Wansu believed that for heat syndromes such as sores and ulcers, moxibustion shouldn't be applied to those with pus or superficial ones. However, it can be used for other types to expel the evils. To treat bone fever, which is a type of deficient heat, moxibustion at Dazhui (GV14), where the bones converge, can be applied.

KNOWLEDGE DATABASE: LITERATURE

***Collection of Writings on the Mechanism of Disease, Suitability of Qi, and the Safeguarding of Life as Discussed in the "Basic Questions" (Sù Wèn Bìng Jī Qì Yí Bǎo Mìng Jí*, 素问病机气宜保命集)**

Collection of Writings on the Mechanism of Disease, Suitability of Qi, and the Safeguarding of Life as Discussed in the "Basic Questions" is a 3-volume comprehensive medical book written by Liu Wansu in 1186 during the Jin Dynasty. The author summarized his clinical experience in this book in his later years.

2.9 *Correct Instructions of Medicine*

Volume 1: Possible Questions on Medicine (*Juàn Yī · Yī Xué Huò Wèn,* 卷一 · 医学或问): Moxibustion for deficiency can support the primary yang with warming fire; moxibustion for excess conditions can disperse excessive evils with heat; moxibustion for cold can restore warmth to the qi; and moxibustion for heat can expel trapped heat qi outward. This illustrates the application of fire to address dryness.

Yu Tuan adopted Zhu Danxi's medical theories, especially Zhu Danxi's comment about moxibustion, which states that "Fire can draw and expel heat and toxin due to its smooth characteristics, representing the application of a contrary treatment". Building on this, Yu Tuan developed a further theoretical summary. He believed that moxibustion could be applied to all types of syndromes, including deficiency, excess, cold, and heat. Specifically, for heat syndromes, moxibustion could help expel the trapped heat qi outward.

3. Note

The theory that "moxibustion is contraindicated in the treatment of heat syndrome" is derived from the concept of fire malpractice in the *Treatise on Cold Damage*. Fire malpractice treatments are not limited to moxibustion but also include other treatments such as the fire needle and the hot compresses. Some doctors of later generations did not thoroughly analyze the concepts of "fire malpractice" and "fire calamity" as described in *Treatise on Cold Damage*, but simply attributed these adverse consequences to moxibustion and proposed that "moxibustion is contraindicated for the treatment of heat syndromes". This opinion doesn't align with clinical practice. As a result, many practitioners continued to document extensive cases of treating heat syndromes with moxibustion and further elaborated on the theory. In fact, the scope of heat syndromes is quite broad. Whether moxibustion can be applied should be determined based on the specific circumstances and cannot be generalized.

Reflections

(1) The idea that "Moxibustion is contraindicated in the treatment of heat syndrome" originated from Zhang Zhongjing's theory of "fire malpractice". Although this idea lacks solid literature and clinical evidence, moxibustion is still rarely used for heat syndromes in modern clinical practice. Are there any other similar phenomena in medical practice?

(2) Can heat syndromes be treated with moxibustion? How can this opinion be verified?

Terms and Synonyms

(1) Fundamentals of T.C.M.

Term	Synonym	Chinese
Syndrome differentiation	• Pattern differentiation • Pattern identification	辨　证
Eight-principle syndrome differentiation	Pattern differentiation by the eight principles	八纲辨证

(2) Book names

Term	Synonym	Chinese
Treatise on Cold Damage and Miscellaneous Diseases	*Shang Han Za Bing Lun*	伤寒杂病论
Treatise on Cold Damage	*Shang Han Lun*	伤寒论

(continued)

Term	Synonym	Chinese
Essentials from the Golden Cabinet	*Jin Gui Yao Lue*	金匮要略
Collection of Writings on the Mechanism of Disease, Suitability of Qi, and the Safeguarding of Life as Discussed in the "Basic Questions"	*Su Wen Bing Ji Qi Yi Bao Ming Ji*	素问病机气宜保命集

(3) Chapters of *The Inner Classic*

The Spiritual Pivot

Term	Synonym	Chinese
Carbuncles and Abscesses	*Yong Ju*	痈 疽

Topic 2

Preventive Moxibustion

1. General introduction to preventive moxibustion

"Preventive treatment" is an important principle in traditional Chinese medicine. In acupuncture and moxibustion, there's a technique known as "preventive acupuncture and moxibustion" or "preventive moxibustion", which involves using acupuncture and moxibustion to prevent illness before it occurs. Moxibustion can warm the body, promote the circulation of qi and blood, and strengthen healthy qi to expel pathogenic factors. As a result, it has been used by practitioners in past dynasties as a preventive measure against diseases. In modern clinical practice, moxibustion is frequently used by non-professionals due to its simplicity, convenience, and effectiveness. It is also being used increasingly for disease prevention and to prevent deterioration.

2. The development of preventive moxibustion

2.1 *The Inner Classic*

The Normal and the Adverse of *The Spiritual Pivot* (*Líng Shū · Nì Shùn*, 灵枢 · 逆顺): Top doctors use needling before the onset of disease, before pathogens become robust; or after pathogens have weakened...Hence the saying that top doctors focus on preventing diseases rather than treating those that have already developed, which precisely reflects this approach.

Major Discussion on the Regulation of Spirit in Four Seasons of *Basic Questions* (*Sù Wèn · Sì Qì Tiáo Shén Dà Lùn*, 素问 · 四气调神大论): Sages focus on preventing diseases rather than treating them, and on preventing disturbances rather than addressing them after they arise. This is exactly the essence of their approach. Treating a disease only after it occurs or addressing a disturbance only after it has happened is akin to digging a well only when you feel thirsty or forging weapons only after a war has broken out. Isn't it too late?

In *The Inner Classic*, the general principle of "preventive treatment" is introduced, highlighting the effectiveness of preventive treatment with acupuncture as an example. However, there're no specific methods for using moxibustion in disease prevention.

KNOWLEDGE DATABASE: LITERATURE

The Normal and The Adverse of *The Spiritual Pivot* (*Líng Shū · Nì Shùn*, 灵枢·逆顺): The 55th chapter of the *Ling Shu*. It emphasizes the importance of early diagnosis and treatment, which should be based on the normal and adverse conditions of qi, the excessive or deficient state of the vessel and the overall disease condition. It also highlights that for diseases, there're three conditions: those that can be treated with needling, those that can't be treated with needling yet, and those that are no longer suitable for needling.

Major Discussion on the Regulation of Spirit in Four Seasons of *Basic Questions* (*Sù Wèn · Sì Qì Tiáo Shén Dà Lùn*, 素问·四气调神大论): The 2nd chapter of *Su Wen*. It primarily discusses how to preserve health and prevent diseases by adapting to the changes in weather throughout the four seasons.

2.2 *Treatise on the Origins and Manifestations of Various Diseases*

Volume 45: Infant Care (*Juàn Sì Shí Wǔ · Yǎng Xiǎo Èr Hòu*, 卷四十五·养小儿候): Be aware that preventive acupuncture and moxibustion should not be applied to healthy newborns... In the region between the Yellow River and the Luo River, which is typically cold, children are prone to convulsions. Consequently, there is a practice of applying preventive moxibustion to 3-day-old newborns to help prevent these issues. Additionally, moxibustion is sometimes applied to the cheek to prevent lockjaw.

Chao Yuanfang from the Sui Dynasty recorded preventive acupuncture and moxibustion, providing detailed accounts of using preventive moxibustion to prevent diseases in newborns. This practice was a form of preventive moxibustion.

2.3 *Important Formulas worth a Thousand Gold Pieces*

> *Volume 29: No. 6, Moxibustion Rules* of *Important Formulas Worth a Thousand Gold Pieces for Emergency*: For individuals who travel to the Wu or Shu regions to serve as officials, frequent moxibustion on two or three areas of the body is necessary, and the resulting wounds should remain unhealed for some time. This practice helps prevent local miasma, pestilence, warm Nue, and toxic qi from affecting people. This is why moxibustion is particularly popular in the Wu and Shu regions.
>
> *Volume 27: No. 10, Bladder Diseases* of *Supplement to "Important Formulas Worth a Thousand Gold Pieces"* (*Qiān Jīn Yì Fāng · Juàn Èr Shí Qī · Pǎng Guāng Bìng Dì Shí*, 千金翼方·卷二十七·膀胱病第十): For vomiting and diarrhea, moxibustion may not provide an immediate cure, but it can help prevent fatal consequences. Preventive moxibustion should not be applied in these cases. Some individuals may initially experience only abdominal pain, while others may have diarrhea followed by vomiting. Moxibustion should be administered according to the specific symptoms. Salt can be placed in the navel for 14 cones of moxibustion, which can also help treat distension and fullness.

Formulas worth a Thousand Gold Pieces describes preventive moxibustion for preventing infectious diseases through suppurative moxibustion. However, the *Supplement to "Important Formulas Worth a Thousand Gold Pieces"* states that for cases of vomiting and diarrhea that don't improve immediately after moxibustion, preventive moxibustion shouldn't be used. Instead, treatment should be tailored to the specific symptoms of the patients.

2.4 *Formulas from Benevolent Sages Compiled during the Taiping Era*

> *Volume 100: Detailed Illustration of 45 Human Figures* (*Juàn Yī Bǎi · Jù Liè Sì Shí Wǔ Rén Xíng*, 卷第一百·具列四十五人形): One to two, or three to five months before a stroke occurs in individuals, there will be a sudden onset of a sour, heavy, and stubborn numb feeling in the feet or legs from time to time, and it will take quite some time before the feeling is alleviated. This is a sign of an impending stroke. In this case, moxibustion should be applied immediately to Sanli (ST36) and Juegu (GB39), with three cones on each of the four points.

In the *Formulas from Benevolent Sages Compiled during the Taiping Era*, moxibustion on Zusanli

(ST36) and Xuanzhong (GB39) for preventing stroke was recorded. This method was later cited in various texts, including *The Great Compendium of Acupuncture and Moxibustion*, and has had a significant influence.

2.5 *The Teachings of Bian Que*

> *Volume 1: Moxibustion Methods from Huangdi*: For persistent fever, which may gradually develop into consumptive diseases in women after childbirth, apply 300 cones of moxibustion immediately to the area below the navel.
>
> *Volume 1: The Necessity of Memorizing Supporting Yang* (*Juàn Shàng · Xū Zhì Fú Yáng*, 卷上·须识扶阳): When people are free from disease, they should apply moxibustion to Guanyuan (CV4), Qihai (CV6), Mingmen (GV4), and Zhongwan (CV12)...Although immortality can't be achieved, a long life of over 100 years can be guaranteed.

Dou Cai recorded the method of preventing consumptive diseases caused by postpartum fever through moxibustion. He also proposed a healthcare moxibustion method aimed at prolonging life.

2.6 *Classic of Nourishing Life with Acupuncture and Moxibustion*

> *Volume 1: 15 Points on the Midline of the Abdomen* (*Juàn Yī · Fù Bù Zhōng Háng Shí Wǔ Zué*, 卷一·腹部中行十五穴): To maintain good health, ensure continuous oozing at Sanli (ST36) and Dantian.
>
> *Volume 3: Deficiency and Impairment* (*Juàn Sān · Xū Sǔn*, 卷三·虚损): The administration of strong tonics can lead to excessive heat in the spleen and stomach, worsening poor appetite... To address this, moxibustion should be applied to Weiwan (CV12).
>
> *Volume 3: Deficiency and Impairment*: Qihai (CV4) is considered the sea of original qi. Original qi is the foundation of the human body; thus, if the original qi is well-preserved, it can protect against diseases. However, if it's depleted, a person may die even in the absence of illness. Therefore, moxibustion should be applied frequently to strengthen the original yang. Waiting to apply moxibustion only after the onset of disease will be too late.
>
> *Volume 3: Deficiency and Impairment*: To strengthen the spleen and stomach, moxibustion should be applied to acupoints, including Pishu (BL20) and Shenshu (BL23).

Wang Zhizhong emphasized the importance of the spleen and stomach. In his book, he described methods for strengthening these organs through moxibustion applied to acupoints such as Pishu (BL20), Shenshu (BL23), Zhongwan (CV12), and others. Besides, he also recorded methods for preventing diseases and prolonging life by applying moxibustion to Qihai (CV4), Dantian, and Zusanli (ST36).

KNOWLEDGE DATABASE: CULTURE

Dantian (丹田)

Dantian, which literally means "fields of pill", originally referred to a concept in Taoist Neidan (internal alchemy, 内丹)—a practice focused on cultivating essence, qi, and shen within the body to achieve immortality. The Dantian is considered the storage place for essence, qi, and shen.

In traditional Chinese medicine, Dantian can refer to specific acupoints located below the navel, such as Qihai (CV6), Shimen (CV5), or Guanyuan (CV4). However, it generally denotes the region below the navel.

2.7 *Pictorial Appendices to "The Classified Classic"*

Volume 8: Points of the Conception Vessel (*Juàn Bā · Rèn Mài Xué*, 卷八 · 任脉穴): Therefore, moxibustion should be applied to Shenque (CV8) after refined salt has been placed inside; and the more cones used, the better. Using three to five hundred cones of moxibustion can not only help cure disease but also prolong life.

In the Ming Dynasty, Zhang Jiebin proposed a method for curing diseases and prolonging life by using salt-insulated moxibustion on Shenque (CV8), as outlined in *Pictorial Appendices to "The Classified Classic"*.

2.8 *Questions and Answers on Acupuncture and Moxibustion*

Volume 3: Acupuncture and moxibustion are considered the last resorts for treating diseases... When moxibustion is applied to a specific point, the surrounding muscle may become hard, resembling nails on a boat. Qi and blood can become stagnated in this area, impairing their flow. There was once a case of a crippled individual with pathogenic factors in the foot Shaoyang meridian. Moxibustion was applied to several points along this meridian, superior to the lateral malleolus. A doctor inserted a needle into Linqi (GB41) to guide the qi to the affected area. However, the qi halted at the moxibustion scar and could not progress further. This led to the understanding that moxa fire could damage the meridians. In emergency situations where it is essential to promote the circulation of qi, there might not be any other choice. When patients suffer from pathogenic invasions in the meridians, there's no alternative but to use moxibustion. Is there any benefit to applying moxibustion to healthy individuals?

In the Ming Dynasty, Wang Ji challenged the practice of preventive moxibustion. He believed that moxibustion could harden the muscles and disrupt the circulation of blood and qi. According to him, using moxibustion on healthy individuals might impair qi and blood circulation in emergency situations, thus he opposed its use during disease-free periods.

3. Note

Acupuncture and moxibustion are both commonly used clinical treatment methods. However, moxibustion is simpler and easier to learn than acupuncture. It's safer to use and does not require complex professional knowledge, making it more accessible to non-professionals. Additionally, its preventive and health-care benefits are widely recognized. Ancient literature indicates that preventive moxibustion has specific indications. However, whether healthy individuals should receive moxibustion in the absence of disease remains a topic of controversy.

Reflections

"Moxibustion during the three-fu periods (the hottest days of summer)" and "natural moxibustion during the three-nine periods (the coldest days of winter)" have become relatively popular treatment methods in recent years. Both use moxibustion (either warming moxibustion or natural moxibustion) to prevent disease and deterioration. What is their documentary basis, and what are the similarities and differences between them? How would you assess these two treatments?

Terms and Synonyms

(1) History, culture and people

Term	Chinese	Explanations
Dantian	丹 田	The area below the navel

(2) Acumox therapeutics

Term	Synonym	Chinese
Preventive treatment	Preventing a disease before it arises	治未病

(3) Chapters of *The Inner Classic*

The Spiritual Pivot

Term	Synonym	Chinese
The Normal and the Adverse	*Ni Shun*	逆 顺

Basic Questions

Term	Synonym	Chinese
Major Discussion on the Regulation of Spirit in Four Seasons	*Si Qi Tiao Shen Da Lun*	四气调神大论

Topic 3

Cold, Heat, Deficiency and Excess in Treatment Principles of Acupuncture and Moxibustion

1. Common understandings of cold, heat, deficiency and excess in the treatment principles of acupuncture and moxibustion

The treatment principles of acupuncture and moxibustion are the fundamental guidelines to follow in acumox treatment. It's determined based on the location and nature of the disease through syndrome differentiation. There are various expressions of the treatment principles in acupuncture and moxibustion, such as reinforcing deficiency and reducing excess, clearing heat and warming cold, treating the root cause of the disease, and adjusting treatment based on the three factors of time, place and person. However, the core principles are succinctly summarized in *The Spiritual Pivot*: "The excess should be reduced, the deficiency should be reinforced, the heat should be treated with swift techniques, the cold should be treated with needle retention, the sinking should be treated with moxibustion, and if it is neither excessive nor deficient, it should be treated according to Jing."

Modern acupuncture texts often reference the treatment principles outlined in *The Spiritual Pivot*, which are typically explained as follows:

"Reinforcing deficiency and reducing excess" involves strengthening the vital qi and expelling pathogenic qi. This approach encompasses three conditions:

- The deficiency should be reinforced, and the sinking should be treated with moxibustion: The deficiency syndromes should be treated with reinforcing techniques along with appropriate acupoints; sinking, which occurs due to qi deficiency, can be treated with moxibustion.
- The excess should be reduced, and the stagnation should be eliminated: The excess syndromes should be treated with reducing techniques and appropriate acupoints; stagnation, which refers to conditions caused by the blockage of blood in the collaterals, can be addressed with blood-letting therapy.
- If it's neither excessive nor deficient, it should be treated according to Jing: For diseases that are neither excessive nor deficient, points on the affected meridian should be selected, and balanced

reinforcing-reducing techniques should be applied.

"Clearing heat and warming cold" is a therapeutic principle targeting diseases with hot and cold properties, respectively. It includes two conditions:

- The heat should be treated with swift techniques: Diseases with a hot property should be addressed with rapid needling and quick withdrawal or by using prick bleeding.
- The cold should be treated with needle retention: Disease with a cold property should be addressed using deep needling and prolonged needle retention.

2. The development of cold, heat, deficiency and excess in treatment principles of acupuncture and moxibustion

2.1 *The Inner Classic*

Nine Needles and Twelve Yuan-Source Points of *The Spiritual Pivot*: To apply the needle, the deficient should be reinforced, the full should be discharged, the stagnation should be eliminated, and the predominance of evils should be reduced.

Explanations of the Small Needle of *The Spiritual Pivot*: The phrase "the deficient should be reinforced" refers to the fact that the condition of weak Qikou should be reinforced. "The full should be discharged", means that the condition of excessive Qikou should be reduced. "The stagnation should be eliminated" refers to removing the blood vessels. "The predominance of evils should be reduced" refers to reducing the excess of pathological factors in each meridian.

Ending and Beginning of *The Spiritual Pivot*: All three vessels pulsate around the big toe, and their excess or deficiency should be assessed. If the deficiency is reduced, it indicates further deficiency, meaning the condition worsens. To needle these vessels, the vessels should be pressed with fingers. If the pulsation is excessive and rapid, it should be reduced immediately; if it is deficient and slow, it should be reinforced. Failure to follow this approach may worsen the condition. Regarding the pulsation, the Yangming is found in the upper part, the Jueyin is in the middle, and the Shaoyin is in the lower part.

The Meridians of *The Spiritual Pivot*: For the treatment of these conditions, the excess should be reduced, the deficiency should be reinforced, the heat should be treated with swift techniques, the cold should be treated with needle retention, the sinking should be treated with moxibustion, and if it is neither excessive nor deficient, it should be treated according to Jing. Excess means that Renying is one time bigger than Cunkou; deficiency means that Renying is smaller than

Cunkou.

Diseases of Cold and Heat of *The Spiritual Pivot*: The foot Taiyang meridian has a branch that enters the cheek and spreads to the teeth, known as Jiaosun. This branch can be used to treat decayed upper teeth through the region anterior to the nose and cheek. When the vessel is affected by disease, it becomes excessive; and excess should be reduced, while deficiency should be reinforced.

Prohibition and Submission of *The Spiritual Pivot* (*Líng Shū · Jìn Fú*, 灵枢 · 禁服): If the Renying pulse being one time bigger than the Cunkou pulse, it indicates a disease in the foot Shaoyang. If it is both larger and rapid, it indicates a disease in the hand Shaoyang. If the Renying pulse is two times larger, it indicates a disease in the foot Taiyang. If it is twice as large and also rapid, the disease is in the hand Taiyang. If the Renying pulse is three times larger, it suggests a disease in the foot Yangming. If it is three times larger and also rapid, the disease is in the hand Yangming. An excessive pulse indicates heat, while a deficient pulse indicates cold. A tight pulse indicates painful obstruction, and a regularly intermittent pulse indicates alternating periods of aggravation and alleviation. The excess should be reduced, while the deficiency should be reinforced. A tight pulse accompanied by pain should be addressed through muscle treatments. A regularly intermittent pulse should be treated with removal of blood collaterals and medicinal decoctions. Sinking conditions should be treated with moxibustion. If the pulse is neither excessive nor deficient, it should be treated according to Jing, which involves a technique known as Jing needling. When the Renying pulse is four times larger, and both large and rapid, it is referred to as "overflowing of yang", which signifies an external yang condition resulting from the repulsion of yin qi. This condition is considered incurable. To diagnose diseases of the zang-fu organs, both the root and the tip of the related meridians should be examined and pressed, and the cold and heat should be assessed. If the Cunkou pulse is one time larger than the Renying pulse, it indicates a disease in the foot Jueyin. If it is one time larger and also rapid, the disease is in the hand pericardium. If the Cunkou pulse is twice as large, the disease is in the foot Shaoyin. If it is twice as large and also rapid, the disease is in the hand Shaoyin. If the Cunkou pulse is three times larger, it suggests a disease in the foot Taiyin; if it is three times larger and also rapid, the disease is in the hand Taiyin. An excessive pulse indicates distension and fullness, cold in the center, and issues with food digestion. A deficient pulse indicates heat in the center, diarrhea, shortness of breath, and changes in urine color. A tight pulse indicates painful obstruction; and a regularly intermittent pulse indicates alternating periods of pain and relief. The excess should be reduced, while the deficiency should be reinforced. For a tight pulse, start with needling and then apply moxibustion. Regularly intermittent pulses should be treated with removal of blood collaterals, followed by regulation. Sinking conditions should be treated with moxibustion only. The sinking condition is caused by the internal coagulation of blood in the vessels. Since the blood is coagulated and cold, moxibustion is recommended. If the pulse is neither excessive nor deficient, treatment should be based on the principles of Jing. When the Cunkou pulse is four times larger, it is referred to as internal closure. If internal closure is both large and rapid, it is considered incurable. To diagnose diseases of the zang-fu organs, both the root and the tip of the related meridians should be inspected and examined to assess for cold and heat conditions...The general principles are as follows: the excessive pulse should be reduced only, while the deficient should be reinforced only. A tight pulse should be treated with moxibustion, acupuncture, and medical decoction. Sinking conditions should be treated with moxibustion only. If the pulse is neither excessive nor deficient, it should be treated according to Jing. Jing treatment refers to the use of medical decoction, as well as moxibustion and acupuncture.

The treatment principle of reinforcing deficiency and reducing excess is derived from the concept "The excess should be reduced, the deficiency should be reinforced" in *The Meridians* of *The Spiritual Pivot*. However, the meanings of these two principles are not entirely identical. The exposition in *The Meridians* originates from the concepts of *Prohibition and Submission*. According to these two chapters, "excess" and "deficiency" here refer not to the excess and deficiency of syndrome, but to the excess and deficiency of pulses. The pulse-taking method involves comparing the Renying and Cunkou pulses. The principle mentioned in *Nine Needles and Twelve Yuan-Source Points* lacks specific context, but from the simultaneous discussion of "the full should be discharged" and "the predominance of evils should be reduced", it appears that "the full should be discharged" doesn't refer to excess syndromes resulting from the predominance of evils. Rather, it and the preceding "the deficient should be reinforced" are very likely from the viewpoint of palpating the meridians or vessels.

In *Prohibition and Submission*, in addition to the principle "the excess should be reduced, while the deficiency should be reinforced", it is also stated that "a tight pulse accompanied by pain should be addressed through muscle treatments. A regularly intermittent pulse should be treated with removal of blood collaterals and medicinal decoctions, and sinking conditions should be treated with moxibustion". These guidelines are derived from palpation, including the diagnosis and examination of the pulses, skin, and muscles of the body. The sentences are followed by "in order to verify diseases of the zang-fu organs, the root and the tip should be examined and pressed, and the cold and heat should be observed". Therefore, the terms "cold", "heat" and "sinking" in *The Meridians* and *Prohibition and Submission* should not be understood merely as cold syndromes, heat syndromes, or sinking of qi due to qi deficiency. Instead, they should be interpreted as symptoms and signs identified through palpation in the areas where the meridians pass.

In addition to determining deficiency and excess using the Renying-Cunkou diagnostic skill, another method involves assessing the forcefulness or weakness of pulsation in a specific area to judge deficiency and excess, as illustrated in *Ending and Beginning* and *Diseases of Cold and Heat*. In *Explanations of the Small Needle*, when discussing the treatment principles in *Nine Needles and Twelve Yuan-Source Points*, it interprets deficiency and excess in relation to the deficiency and excess of Qikou, specifically referring to the vessel of Cunkou.

Regarding the phrase "being treated according to Jing" for cases that are "neither excessive nor deficient", in *Prohibition and Submission*, "Jing" doesn't refer to the meridians but means "common", implying the use of common therapies. Specifically, it refers to "Jing treatment", which includes medical decoction as well as moxibustion and acupuncture, as detailed in the following text of *Prohibition and Submission.*

Regarding the principles of "The stagnation should be eliminated, and the predominance of evils should be reduced" in *Nine Needles and Twelve Yuan-Source Points*, *Explanations of the Small Needle* explains them as "removing blood vessels" and "reducing the excess of pathological factors in each meridian". The latter connected the excess of each meridian with evil qi, thereby introducing the concept of deficiency and excess in pathogenesis. This indicates that the idea that "predominance of evil qi indicates excess while deprived essence qi indicates deficiency" is integrated into the therapeutic principles of acupuncture in *The Inner Classic*.

KNOWLEDGE DATABASE: LITERATURE

Prohibition and Submission of *The Spiritual Pivot* (*Líng Shū · Jìn Fú*, 灵枢 · 禁服): The 48th chapter of the *Ling Shu*. It discusses the need to follow the circulation of the meridians and its relation to wei qi. Diseases can be diagnosed by observing the pulses at Renying and Cunkou. The chapter also discusses how moxibustion, needling, or medication can be applied according to the different properties of diseases.

KNOWLEDGE DATABASE: CULTURE

Different meanings of Jing (经) and Polysemy of Chinese Characters

The character Jing (经) is frequently used in Chinese, as seen in terms such as meridians (经脉), classics (经典), manage (经营), endure (经受), pass through (经过) and common (经常). This phenomenon, where one character has multiple meanings, is a typical feature of the Chinese language and is known as polysemy.

In modern Chinese, the meaning of a character is usually easy to identify because modern Chinese often uses multi-character words to clarify different meanings. However, in classical Chinese, it is common for a single character to convey multiple meanings, which must be inferred from the context. This can be challenging for readers and often requires specialized training.

Take the use of "Jing" in the treatment principle mentioned above as an example. In this translation, its pinyin is used instead of specifying its meanings, because there're two different interpretations of this character. Most modern explanations of these treatment principles are based on misunderstandings that have persisted for over a thousand years. To clarify the principles, it's necessary to use pinyin rather than relying directly on either of the two interpretations.

2.2 *The Classic of Questioning*

The 69th Issue (Liù Shí Jiǔ Nàn, 六十九难): In *The Classic*, it's stated that the excess should be reduced, the deficiency should be reinforced, and if the condition is neither excessive nor deficient, it should be treated according to Jing. What does this mean?

This is the answer: For the deficiency, the Mother should be reinforced; for the excess, the Son should be reduced. Reinforcing techniques should be applied before reducing techniques. When it is said that "if the condition is neither excessive nor deficient, it should be treated according to Jing", it means that the disease originates from the meridian itself rather than from external pathogens. Therefore, treatment should focus on the meridian itself, which is why it's said to be "treated according to Jing".

In *The Classic of Questioning*, the original meanings of deficiency and excess in *The Inner Classic* are not explored in depth. Instead, the concept that "the excess should be reduced, the deficiency should be reinforced" is explained as a technique of reinforcing and reducing. This interpretation represents a reinforcing-reducing approach developed from the combination of the five-phase doctrine and the five transport points theory. This interpretation will facilitate the understanding of deficiency and excess in the common aspect of pathogenesis.

Moreover, regarding "be treated according to Jing", *The Classic of Questioning* held that if a disease is caused by the meridian itself without the involvement of external evils, it should be treated with the meridian itself. This theory was later supported by Yang Shangshan, Ma Shi, and Zhang Jiebin, and it had a significant and widespread influence.

KNOWLEDGE DATABASE: LITERATURE

The 69th Issue of *The Classic of Questioning* (*Nàn Jīng · Liù Shí Jiǔ Nàn,* 难经 · 六十九难): The 69th issue of *The Classic of Questioning.* It introduces the principles of Mother-Son reinforcing and reducing techniques.

KNOWLEDGE DATABASE: PEOPLE

Ma Shi (马莳)

Ma Shi, with the courtesy name Zhonghua (仲化) and the literary names Xuantai (玄台) or Yuantai (元台), was a famous medical practitioner of the Ming Dynasty. He was born in the 15th century and passed away in the 16th century.

Ma Shi's most notable contribution is his annotation and compilation of *The Inner Classic* into two books: *Annotation, Review and Elaboration on The Spiritual Pivot of Huangdi's Inner Classic* (*Huáng Dì Nèi Jīng Líng Shū Zhù Zhèng Fā Wēi,* 黄帝内经灵枢注证发微) and *Annotation, Review and Elaboration on Basic Questions of Huangdi's Inner Classic* (*Huáng Dì Nèi Jīng Sù Wèn Zhù Zhèng Fā Wēi,* 黄帝内经素问注证发微). Compiled in 1586, these works are comprehensive annotated versions of *The Spiritual Pivot* and *Basic Questions*, with the one on *The Spiritual Pivot* being the earliest.

2.3 *Replenished and Supplementarily Annotated Basic Questions of Huangdi's Inner Classic* (*Chóng Guǎng Bǔ Zhù Huáng Dì Nèi Jīng Sù Wèn,* 重广补注黄帝内经素问)

Discussion on Jue Syndrome (*Jué Lùn,* 厥论): If it's neither excessive nor deficient, it should be treated according to Jing. "Neither excessive nor deficient" means that the evil qi is not exuberant and the vital qi is not weakened. In such cases, treatment can follow standard methods, including acupoints, needle retention and breathing techniques.

When explaining the sentence "If it's neither excessive nor deficient, it should be treated according to Jing" in *Discussion on Jue Syndrome* of *Basic Questions*, Wang Bing interpreted "deficient" and "excessive" as referring to the deficiency and excess of pathogenesis. As for "being treated according to Jing", he believed it meant to determine the treatment approach based on the standard guidelines for acupoints. This perspective was later adopted by Hua Shou.

KNOWLEDGE DATABASE: LITERATURE

Replenished and Supplementarily Annotated Basic Questions of Huangdi's Inner Classic (Chóng Guǎng Bǔ Zhù Huáng Dì Nèi Jīng Sù Wèn, 重广补注黄帝内经素问)

In 762 during the Tang Dynasty, Wang Bing annotated the *Basic Questions from Huangdi's Inner Classic* based on the edition of Quan Yuanqi, a physician from the Sui Dynasty, and supplemented the lost seventh volume with seven chapters of "major discussion". Between 1027 and 1067, the book was collated and renamed "*Replenished and Supplementarily Annotated Basic Questions of Huangdi's Inner Classic*", and was subsequently published and finalized.

KNOWLEDGE DATABASE: LITERATURE

Discussion on Jue Syndrome of *Basic Questions* (*Sù Wèn · Jué Lùn*, 素问·厥论): The 45th chapter of the *Su Wen*. It mainly introduces the causes, pathogenesis, classification, and manifestations of jue syndrome.

2.4 *Formulas from Benevolent Sages Compiled during the Taiping Era*

> *Volume 99*: When using acupuncture, it is essential to understand the acupoints, reinforce the deficient, reduce the excessive, disperse the hard, aid the soft, and modify the tight and the moderate. This approach ensures a constant flow of the ying qi and wei qi, and not to violate the principle. As stated in *The Classic*: The excess should be reduced, the deficiency should be reinforced, and if it's neither excessive nor deficient, it should be treated according to Jing. However, for deficiency, the Mother should be reinforced; while for excess, the Son should be reduced. Reinforcing techniques should be applied before reducing techniques. "If it's neither excessive nor deficient, it should be treated according to Jing", meaning that the disease originates from the meridian itself rather than from external pathogens. Therefore, treatment should focus on the meridian itself, which is why it's said to be "treated according to Jing".

In later texts, the terms "excess" and "deficiency" in the acumox principle of "the excess should be reduced, the deficiency should be reinforced" are typically understood as referring to the deficiency and excess of pathogenesis. The 99th volume of *Formulas from Benevolent Sages Compiled during the Taiping Era* is a case that combines the acupuncture principles elaborated in *Important Formulas Worth a Thousand Gold Pieces for Emergency* and *The Classic of Questioning.* These elaborations typically discussed the acumox principles without reference to pulse diagnosis. This not only reflects a certain misapprehension of acumox principles at that time, but also intensifies the misunderstanding among later practitioners. In modern textbooks, concepts such as cold, heat, deficiency, excess, and sinking are all explained as syndromes, largely based on these misunderstandings.

3. Note

The treatment principles of acumox in *The Inner Classic*—"The excess should be reduced, the deficiency should be reinforced, the heat should be treated with swift techniques, the cold should be treated with needle retention, the sinking should be treated with moxibustion, and if it is neither excessive nor deficient, it should be treated according to Jing" —were originally based on meridian-collateral palpation. The modern understanding of this principle has deviated from palpation, leading to a misunderstanding of the acumox principles in *The Inner Classic*. This misinterpretation also hinders the correct understanding of other theories and methods in *The Inner Classic*.

Reflections

The principle "The excess should be reduced, the deficiency should be reinforced, the heat should be treated with swift techniques, the cold should be treated with needle retaining, the sinking should be treated with moxibustion, and if it's neither excessive nor deficient, it should be treated according to Jing" can be applied based on either the deficiency and excess of the pulse or the deficiency and excess of the pathogenesis. What are the similarities and differences in treatment decision-making and clinical manipulation between them?

Terms and Synonyms

(1) History, culture and people

Term	Chinese	Explanations
Polysemy	一词多义	One character has various meanings
Ma Shi	马　莳	A famous medical doctor in the Ming Dynasty, the author of *Annotation, Review and Elaboration on The Spiritual Pivot of Huangdi's Inner Classic* and *Annotation, Review and Elaboration on Basic Questions of Huangdi's Inner Classic*
Ma Zhonghua	马仲化	
Ma Xuantai	马玄台	
Ma Yuantai	马元台	

(2) Book names

Term	Synonym	Chinese
Annotation, Review and Elaboration on The Spiritual Pivot of Huangdi's Inner Classic	*Huang Di Nei Jing Ling Shu Zhu Zheng Fa Wei*	黄帝内经 灵枢注证发微
Annotation, Review and Elaboration on Basic Questions of Huangdi's Inner Classic	*Huang Di Nei Jing Su Wen Zhu Zheng Fa Wei*	黄帝内经 素问注证发微
Replenished and Supplementarily Annotated Basic Questions of Huangdi's Inner Classic	*Chong Guang Bu Zhu Huang Di Nei Jing Su Wen*	重广补注 黄帝内经素问

(3) Chapters of *The Inner Classic*

The Spiritual Pivot

Term	Synonym	Chinese
Prohibition and Submission	*Jin Fu*	禁 服

Basic Questions

Term	Synonym	Chinese
Discussion on Jue Syndrome	*Jue Lun*	厥 论

(4) Issues of *The Classic of Questioning*

Term	Pinyin & Chinese	Main Contents
The 69th Issue	*Liu Shi Jiu Nan* 六十九难	Therapeutic principles of acupuncture

Bibliography

1. The Collation Group of Silk Books from Mawangdui Han Tombs. Formulas for Fifty-two Diseases of Silk Books from Mawangdui Han Tombs[M]. Beijing: Cultural Relics Publishing House, 1979.

2. The Collation Group of Bamboo-slip Books from No. 247 Zhangjiashan Han Tomb. Bamboo Slips from Zhangjiashan Han Tombs [Tomb No. 247][M]. Beijing: Cultural Relics Publishing House, 2006.

3. Liang Fanrong. Revealing the Secret of Posthumous Work of Bi Xi and the Lacquer Man[M]. Chengdu: Sichuan Science and Technology Press, 2016.

4. Anonymous. The Classic of Spiritual Pivot[M]. Photocopy of the Zhaofujujingtang block-printed edition in the Ming Dynasty. Beijing: People's Medical Publishing House, 1956.

5. Wang Bing. Replenished and Supplementarily Annotated Basic Questions of Huangdi[M/DK]. Re-block-printed Song Dynasty edition. [Place of publication unknown]: Gu Congde, 1550 (the 29th year of Jiajing era).

6. Wang Jiusi. Collected Annotations to The Classic of Questioning[M/DK]. Block-printed edition. Jinshan: Qian's Shoushan Pavilion Series, 1852 (the second year of Xianfeng era).

7. Huang Longxiang. Compilation and Collation of The Classic of Bright Hall Theory of Huangdi[M]. Beijing: China Medical Science and Technology Press, 1988.

8. Huangfu Mi. The Systematic Classic of Acupuncture and Moxibustion[M]. Photocopy of Yitong Zhengmai edition of the Ming Dynasty. Beijing: People's Medical Publishing House, 1956.

9. Ge Hong. Emergency Formulas to Keep Up One's Sleeve[M/DK]. Block-printed edition. [Place of publication unknown]: Liu Zihua, 1574 (the second year of Wanli era).

10. Yang Shangshan. The Classified Bright Hall Theory of Huangdi's Inner Classic[M/DK]//Liao Ping. The Classified Bright Hall Theory of Huangdi of the Sui Dynasty. Chengdu: Cungu Book Company, 1916.

11. Sun Simiao. Important Formulas Worth a Thousand Gold Pieces for Emergency[M]. Photocopy of the Edo Medicine Photocopy of the Northern Song Dynasty edition. Beijing: People's Medical Publishing House, 1955.

12. Sun Simiao. Supplement to "Important Formulas worth a Thousand Gold Pieces"[M]. Photocopy of the re-block-printed edition in the Qing Dynasty of Meixi Academy edition in the Dade era of the Yuan Dynasty.

Beijing: People's Medical Publishing House, 1955.

13. Wang Tao. Arcane Essentials from the Imperial Library[M]. Photocopy of Jing Yu House's block-printed edition in the 13th year of Chongzhen era of the Ming Dynasty. Beijing: People's Medical Publishing House, 1955.

14. Wang Huaiyin, et al. Formulas from Benevolent Sages Compiled during the Taiping Era[M]. Organized edition. Beijing: People's Medical Publishing House, 1958.

15. Wang Weiyi. Newly Block-Printed Supplementarily Annotated Illustrated Classic of Acupoints on the Bronze Figure[M]. Photocopy of Liu's Yuhaitang edition in the Xuantong era of the Qing Dynasty. Beijing: People's Medical Publishing House, 1955.

16. Zhuang Chuo. The Bright Hall Moxibustion Classic of Xi Fang Zi, Moxibustion Techniques for Gaohuangshu[M]. Li Ding, Wu Zidong, collating and annotating. Shanghai: Shanghai College of Traditional Chinese Medicine Press, 1989.

17. Dou Cai. The Teachings of Bian Que[M]. Li Xiaolu, Yu Zhenxuan, collating. Beijing: Traditional Chinese Medicine Ancient Books Publishing House, 1992.

18. Wang Zhizhong. Classic of Nourishing Life with Acupuncture and Moxibustion[M]. Photocopy of the edition from Wenyuange's Complete Library in the Four Branches of Literature. Beijing: China Bookstore Publishing House, 1987.

19. Wenren Qinian, Sun Juqing. Moxibustion for Emergency[M]. Photocopy of the Shi Ban Tong Xin Lan House' edition from the 16th year of Guangxu era. Beijing: People's Medical Publishing House, 1955.

20. Yan Mingguang, Dou Mo. Collection of Annotations to "Acupuncture Classic on Noon-Midnight Ebb-Flow" and "A Guide to Acupuncture Classics"[M]. Li Ding, Wang Luozhen, Li Lei, commenting and annotating. Shanghai: Shanghai Scientific & Technical Publishers, 1998.

21. Hua Shou. Elucidation on Fourteen Channels [M]//Huang Longxiang. A Collection of Classics on Acupuncture. Beijing: Huaxia Publishing House, 1996.

22. Xu Feng. The Complete Compendium of Acupuncture and Moxibustion[M]. Beijing: People's Medical Publishing House, 1958.

23. Gao Wu. A Collection of Gems in Acupuncture and Moxibustion[M]. Shanghai: Shanghai Scientific & Technical Publishers, 1961.

24. Wang Ji. Questions and Answers on Acupuncture and Moxibustion[M]. Shanghai: Shanghai Scientific & Technical Publishers, 1959.

25. Li Chan. Introduction to Medicine[M]. Tian Daihua, Jin Li, He Shui, Dian Xiao. Tianjin: Tianjin Science and Technology Press, 1999.

26. Yang Jizhou. The Great Compendium of Acupuncture and Moxibustion[M]. Beijing: People's Medical Publishing House, 1963.

27. Wu Qian, et al. Imperial Compilation of Golden Mirror of the Medical Tradition[M]. Third edition. Beijing: People's Medical Publishing House, 1998.

28. Cheng Dan'an. Updated Acupuncture and Moxibustion Therapy in China[M]. Shanghai: Chinese Acupuncture Research Society, 1933.

Index

Acumox Techniques

Acumox Therapeutics

Books

Culture and Others

Fundamentals of T.C.M.

History

Meridians and Points

People

www.ingramcontent.com/pod-product-compliance
Lightning Source LLC
Chambersburg PA
CBHW041754220926
51847CB00014B/205
* 9 7 8 7 5 4 7 8 7 1 9 1 1 *